Radiological Reporting in Clinical Practice

Francesco Schiavon • Fabio Grigenti

Radiological Reporting in Clinical Practice

With a contribution by
Nick van Terheyden

and the collaboration of
Riccardo Berletti
Matteo Costa
Massimo Favat
Manuel Fontana

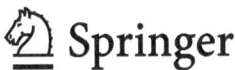 Springer

Authors:
Francesco Schiavon
Radiology Department
San Martino Hospital
Belluno, Italy

Fabio Grigenti
Philosophy Department
University of Padoa
Padoa, Italy

Contributor:
Nick van Terheyden
Director Clinical Advocates,
Philips Health Care Informatics
and Chief Medical Officer,
Philips Speech Recognition
Systems
Laytonsville, MD, USA

Collaborators:
Riccardo Berletti, Matteo Costa, Massimo Favat, Manuel Fontana
Radiology Department, San Martino Hospital, Belluno, Italy

Library of Congress Control Number: 2007940888

ISBN 978-88-470-0681-2 Springer Milan Berlin Heidelberg New York
ISBN 978-88-470-0682-9 (eBook)

Springer is a part of Springer Science+Business Media

© Springer-Verlag Italia 2008

springer.com

Cover design: Simona Colombo, Milan, Italy
Typesetting: C & G di Cerri e Galassi, Cremona, Italy

Springer-Verlag Italia S.r.l. – Via Decembrio 28 – I-20137 Milan

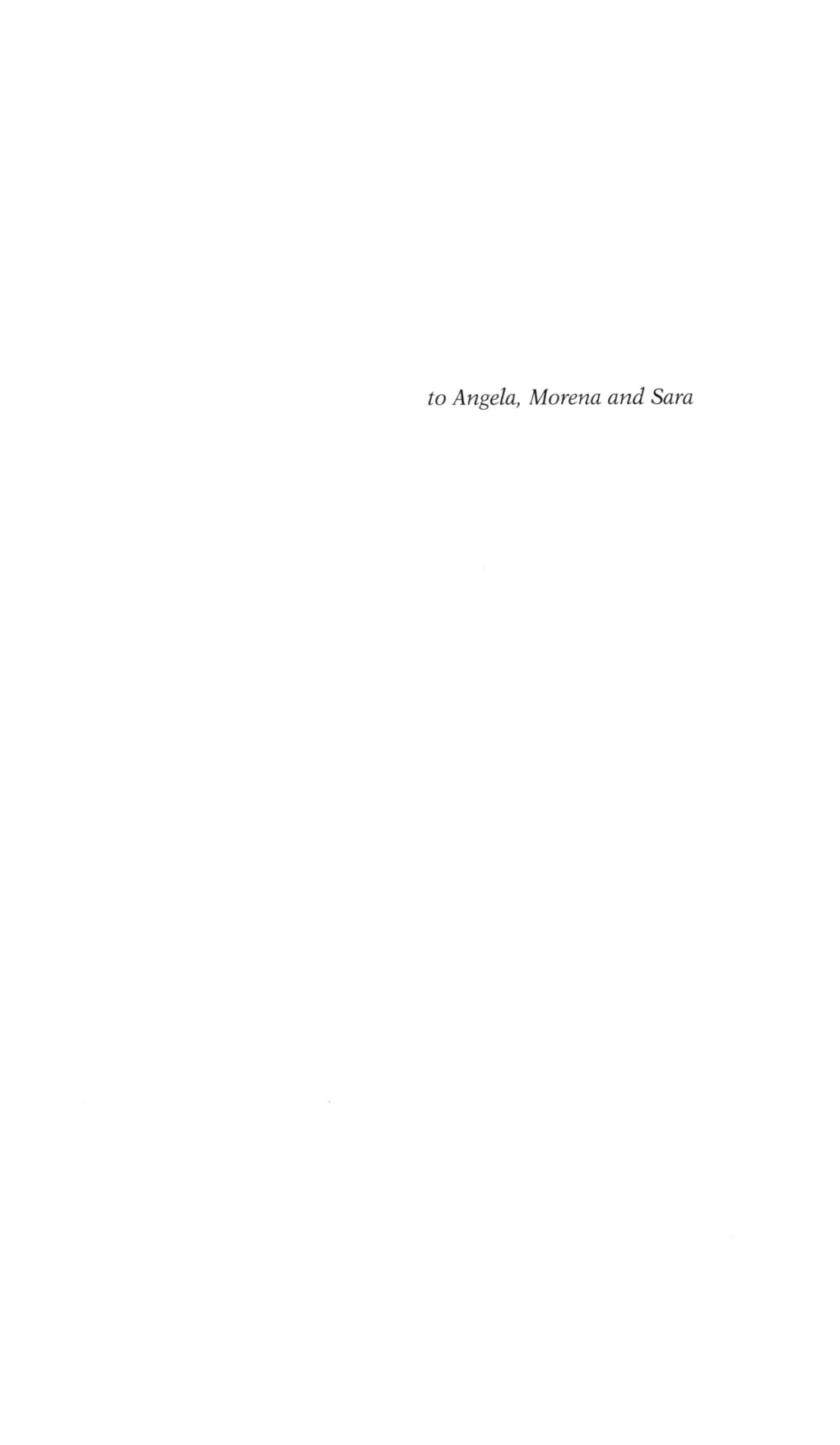

to Angela, Morena and Sara

Note of Thanks

I wish to thank many people, without all of whom I would not have achieved this goal. In chronological order.

First of all, coauthor and friend, Fabio Grigenti, because many years ago he confirmed that this was a good topic, enabling me to gain knowledge and improve, measuring me against himself, giving me ideas and inspiration, and confidently sticking with me on this adventure.

Then, all my medical and technical colleagues, in particular, Riccardo Berletti, Matteo Costa, Massimo Favat, and Manuel Fontana, because – full of admirable enthusiasm and intelligence – they first understood the spirit and aims of this work. They then made their former and continuing experience available to me to the extent that all the iconography presented herein – images and reports – comes from our department.

Also, Antonella Cerri and Alessandra Born from the publishers, Springer: the former because she believed in my project and sponsored it with passion and conviction; the latter because she followed us step by step in the completion of this publication.

Finally, Springer, because they guided me with their famed know-how, giving the work a more apt editorial appearance.

For me, a radiologist working in a medium-sized facility on the periphery of the Italian experience, it is with great honor and pride that – with the assistance of this excellent collaboration and the extensive knowledge gained in my everyday working life – I have written and completed a project that I so deeply desired to undertake.

Francesco Schiavon

Preface

This book is the result of an ambitious goal: to encourage discussion of reporting within two often distant areas – medical and scientific knowledge, and humanistic and philosophical learning. Nowadays, this point of view may seem presumptuous and perhaps even unnecessary. However, it is actually only the rediscovery of an ancient tradition: today, the two disciplines, medicine and philosophy, are different and separate. Historically, they were very closely linked in the *curricula studiorum* and in professional practice. Physicians had to know the basics of literary knowledge, rhetoric, and philosophical philosophy; likewise, philosophers could not ignore the progress made by scientists in their respective fields of research. This was especially true for medicine, the only natural science that was explicitly aimed at humankind and was – and still is – the object of the humanistic culture. Yet the combination we are attempting to implement through this book is justified for another reason, one related to the specific theme of this work: radiological reporting.

Writing the radiologic report is the moment when the radiologist's work is brought together and presented in its final synthesis. The images viewed must ultimately become public in the form of a note of communication written for third parties: the prescribing physician – clinicians in general – and the patient. Here, the specific technical competencies must be accompanied by the sensitivity, culture, and reporting capacities of the radiologist.

People called upon to write a report are not always aware of the technical and logical and conceptual processes governing the operations being carried out: viewing and interpreting the image, putting sense into words, and writing the final draft of the report. This is mainly due to excessive specialization and subdivision of the subjects studied. Obviously, the dynamics of these operations can be understood and controlled by examination approaches and disciplines that often do not directly pertain to the good radiologist's know-how. So, here we attempt to make an initial contribution toward that end.

And we have a further goal. We are convinced that the report is not just a description, a simple continuation of the job of interpreting the radiological image. Inasmuch as it is a document for communicating to others, it has consequences that may, as do all human actions, be evaluated in terms of damages or benefits. Poor communication can cause incomprehension and delays in action, which could be truly harmful; on the other hand, a clear description and effective use of words is often the beginning of a virtuous healthcare procedure.

In other words, whereas the radiological report certainly expresses the physician's knowledge, experience, and capacity, it primarily reflects the physician's responsibility.

November 2007   Francesco Schiavon
                                             Fabio Grigenti

Contents

Chapter 1
Introduction

The radiological report is the medical document that qualifies the radiologist as a clinician and as a specialist, because through it, the radiologist expresses his or her professionalism. Said differently, the report is the radiologist's drug, as will be explained herein.

There is nothing more debatable than the report and how it should be written. It is conditioned by many – perhaps too many – variables that derive from the widest variety of sensitivities and personal and local cultures; also – and more simply – there has never been a specific school in which these rules are taught.

To be of good quality, a report must satisfy some basic requirements. First, it should affect how treatment is handled, outlining its general setup and amending or confirming it when considered necessary (Fig. 1). If a report does not fulfill these functions, either it is the product of a lack of professionalism or it is the response to an unnecessarily requested examination. The report is the quintessential communication tool of the radiologist and is used to describe the results of the radiologist's examination. If the radiologist does not want to irreparably compromise the efficacy of the examination, he or she must be a good interpreter of the images as well as a good communicator. Therefore, a good report:

1. Is effective from the communication point of view, because it utilizes an incisive and adequate structure, form, and vocabulary. To achieve this, the terminology required must comply with all the rules of communication and convey ex-

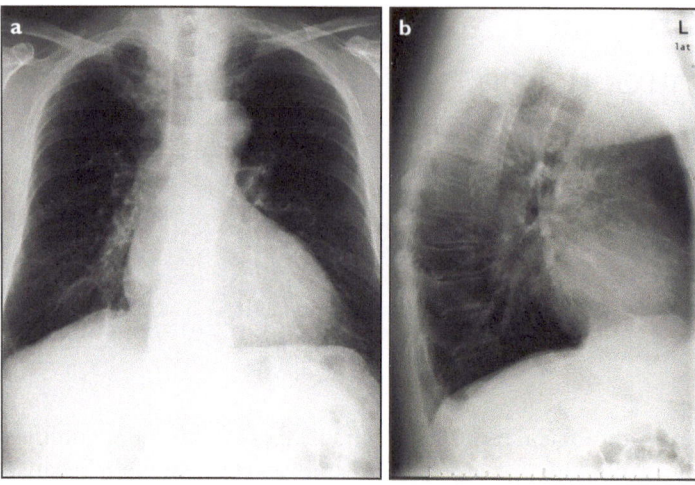

c

[...] The clinical picture described above suggests an initial congestion of the lesser circulation due to insufficiency of the left heart and a consultation with the specialist in cardiology is therefore recommended.

Fig. 1 a-c. Report that has a positive effect on the definition of the clinical situation. The radiological examination of the thorax (**a, b**) is requested because of a "persistent cough": the signs of congestion of the pulmonary circulation resulting from insufficiency of the left heart are described (**c**), and the patient is referred to a competent specialist

actly the radiological interpretation to the prescribing physician (Fig. 2).

2. Respects elementary language rules (grammar, syntax, punctuation, *consecutio temporum*) and must not include any errors caused by inattentiveness. The tools needed to achieve this are the right amount of sensitivity, good knowledge, and adequate information technology support.

3. Avoids, or keeps to a minimum, both interpretation errors ("universal" errors caused by inexperience: "we all make mistakes") and – or even above all – errors caused by carelessness ("individual" errors, caused by negligence: "only people who are not careful make mistakes") (Fig. 3) (Also refer to the chapter "Errors in Reporting").

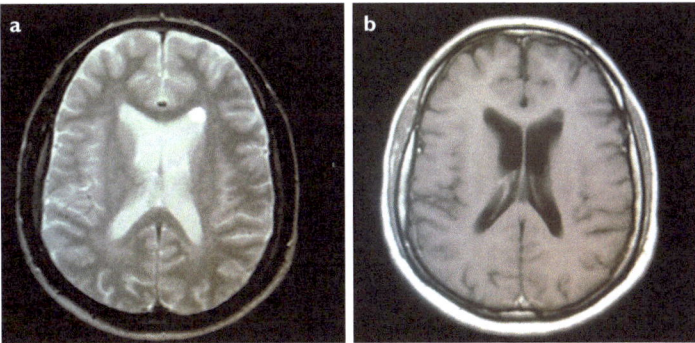

c [...] There is a small round formation with clear margins which projects in the frontal horn of the left lateral ventricle. Said formation shows a signal slightly hyperintense to liquor in all sequences, without any enhancement following the gadolinium. [...] The incidental finding described above is probably connected to a neuroepithelial cyst (ependymal cyst).

Fig. 2 a-c. A small lesion is described – probably an ependymal cyst – indicating its modest clinical impact. **a** Basic T2-weighted sequence. **b** T1-weighted sequence after gadolinium. **c** Report resulting in in effective communication

4. Complies with the increasingly relevant economic constraints found in health care: i.e., the report must not lead to needless expenses – for example, requesting further examinations or checks when these are not necessary and when they solely reflect the inadequacy of the report writer (Fig. 4).

Today, all diagnostic documents must comply with the evidence-based medicine standard. This not only means that the invasiveness of the radiological examination that is requested and carried out – whatever it may be – must be acceptable when related to the clinical problem but that the report must not leave out any qualifying elements of that examination. In fact, it must enhance the value of all the elements (Fig. 5). Basically, just as the request for radiological examination must only be for the strictly necessary and the consequent examination performed as appropriately as possible, likewise, the report must satisfy all clinical requirements stated by the prescribing physician.

a
The examination is requested for suspected pleuritis with dyspnea and pain. No pulmonary lesions. No pleural effusion. Heart is within the limits of normally.

b
[...] Accentuation of bronchovascular pattern in parahilar region of the left upper lobe. No lesions elsewhere. [...]

c
Big hiloparahilar lesion that infiltrates pulmonary artery [...]

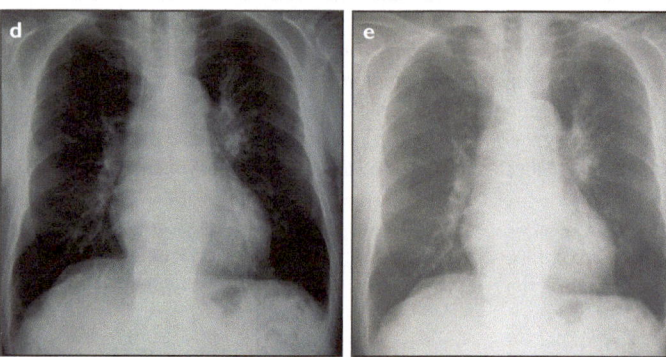

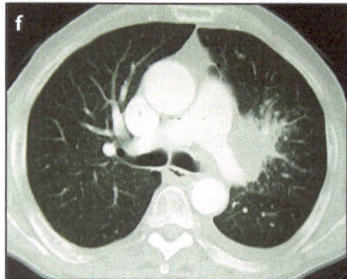

Fig. 3 a-f. Medical reports: thorax X-rays from the first examination, (**a**) second examination (**b**) thorax computed tomography (CT) from the third examination (**c**). **d** Frontal radiograph from the first examination. **e** Frontal radiograph from the second examination. **f** CT scan with contrast medium, "window" for lung, from the third examination.

"Universal" and "individual" errors (see text). Two radiological examinations of a patient's chest (**d, e**), done at a distance of a few months, reported by the same physician. In the second examination (**e**), the physician does not quote the first examination ("individual" error). In neither report does he or she recognize the direct and indirect signs of the subobstructive neoplasia of the trunk of the left upper lobe ("universal" error, although major)

a
Liver presenting an echostructure slightly and diffusively inhomogeneous, likely due to the results of radiotherapy.
[...] The spleen is within the limits for dimensions, diffusively inhomogeneous in a picture of uncertain interpretation (is it because of past radiotherapy?). [...]

b
[...] to better define the hepatic and splenic alterations evident in a previous echography dated 19/02/07 in an LH in remission".

Fig. 4 a, b. The uncertainties expressed by the radiologist could lead to the carrying out of further tests. In this case, as there are the consequences of a Hodgkin's lymphoma, the medical report of the hepatic echography (**a**) creates uncertainty and leads the doctor who requested it to recommend a new control test (CT of the abdomen) to clarify the situation (physician's request) (**b**). With the agreement of the doctor prescribing the test, the CT examination was later changed to a new echography, the results of which were completely negative

As can be seen, a good report entails many requirements that are not always acknowledged, whether taken individually or collectively, each of which may jeopardize the overall report quality.

One of the principal characteristics of current diagnostic imaging is its complex nature due to the number of images and the quantity of information that each one provides. In the past – even in the quite recent past – documentation was never very complete, although at times enriched with some "special" examination (Fig. 6). There were few details in each image, and these could not be modified, being interpreted according to classic semiotic standards. Today, the situation is different: many examinations consist of hundreds of images, as in the case of any multidetector computed tomography (MDCT) scan and high-field magnetic resonance (MR). For these examinations, and even for others consisting of very few images, the images can be manipulated on the screen until they are radically transformed into images with new particulars. There is also an increasingly widespread use of integrated imaging – for example, positron emission tomography (PET) CT – that gathers together all the details and compares them. This function creates new interpretative requirements that derive from

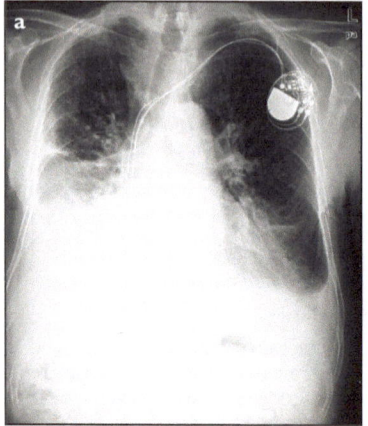

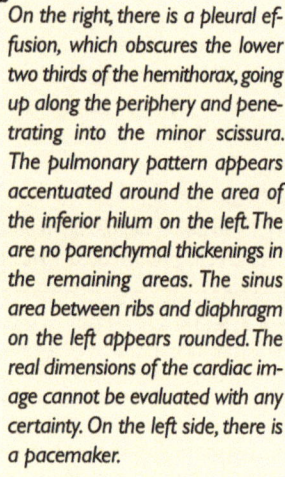

b
On the right, there is a pleural effusion, which obscures the lower two thirds of the hemithorax, going up along the periphery and penetrating into the minor scissura. The pulmonary pattern appears accentuated around the area of the inferior hilum on the left. The are no parenchymal thickenings in the remaining areas. The sinus area between ribs and diaphragm on the left appears rounded. The real dimensions of the cardiac image cannot be evaluated with any certainty. On the left side, there is a pacemaker.

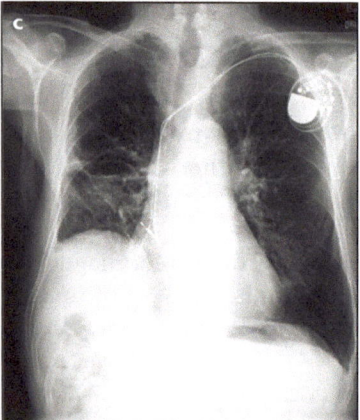

d
Control of previous congestive heart failure.
Compared to the previous test carried out on...., the almost complete regression of the bilateral pleural effusion that was present then can be observed, with reduction on the strengthening of the vascular pattern and on the enlargement of the heart. [...]

Fig. 5 a-d. The reports must respect evidence-based medicine standards. Two reports of wo radiological examinations of the chest (**a, c**) performed on the same patient at an interval of 1 month. **b** First report of little use. **d** Second report is a good medical report

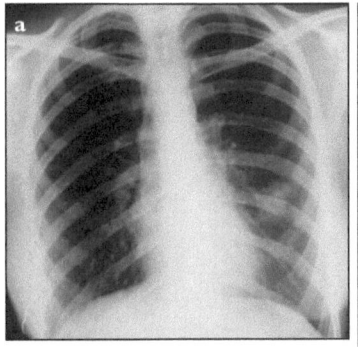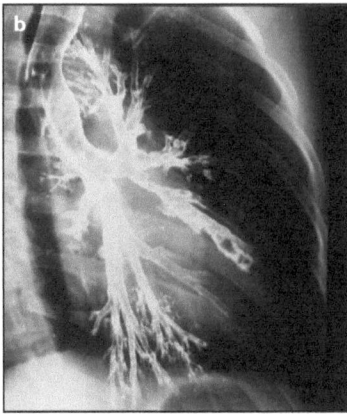

Fig. 6 a, b. Radiological examination of the chest (**a**) and Bronchograph (**b**). During the analogue era, what little information there are was, was of great value. Case of bronchiectasis of the lingula and – to a lesser extent – of the left inferior lobe

the integration of morphological and functional data (Fig. 7). Furthermore, we should also mention examinations – as in the case of the oncology sector – in which two long series of images are compared to evaluate the evolution of the known pathology. And this situation will grow more complicated in the future if Eliot Siegel's prophecy comes true. According to Siegel, at this rate, by 2015, each radiologist will have to evaluate approximately 600,000 images a day.

With the advent of digital technology and the possibility of varying the gray levels of the acquired images on the screen, the power of contrast resolution in space and time has increased so greatly that the human eye is no longer sufficient to see minimum alterations. Therefore, assistance from the computer is required [computer-assisted diagnosis (CAD)]. This is opposite of what once took place with analog images in which, if anything, the problem consisted of not leaving out any lesions due to a defect in acquisition technique, which could not be recovered in any way. Therefore, with advancement from analogical to digital technology and clinical use of high-performance machinery – such as MDCT, high-field MR, and PET CT – the characteristics of imaging have radically changed in a short period of time.

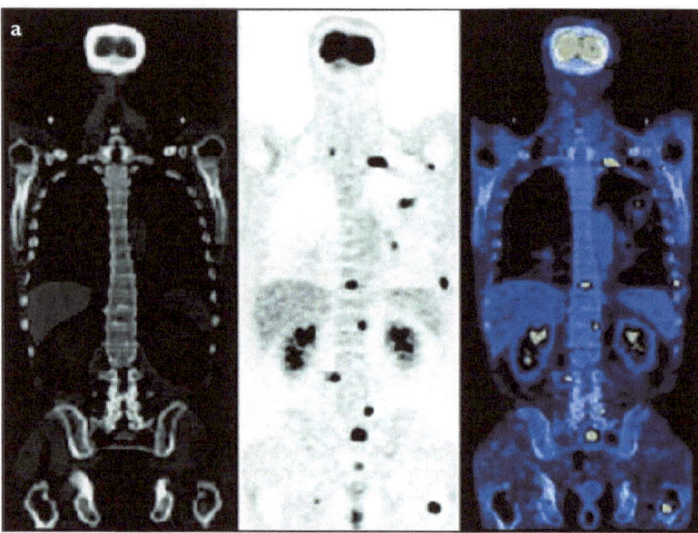

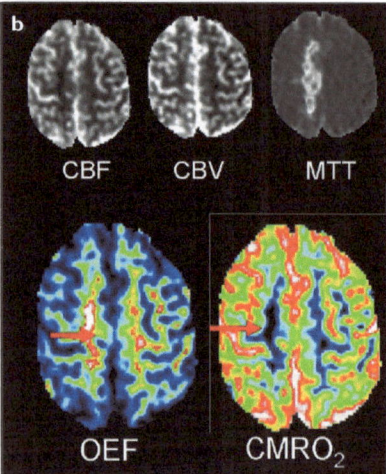

Fig. 7 a, b. Positron emission tomography computed tomography (PET-CT) (**a**). Functional magnetic resonance imaging (MRI). *CBF* cerebral blood flow, *CBV* cerebral blood volume, *MTT* mean transit time, *OEF* oxygen extraction fraction, *CMRO$_2$* cerebral metabolic rate oxygen (**b**). In the pan-explorative and totipotent digital era, information can be excessive and redundant, and it may be necessary to select and hierarchize the reports

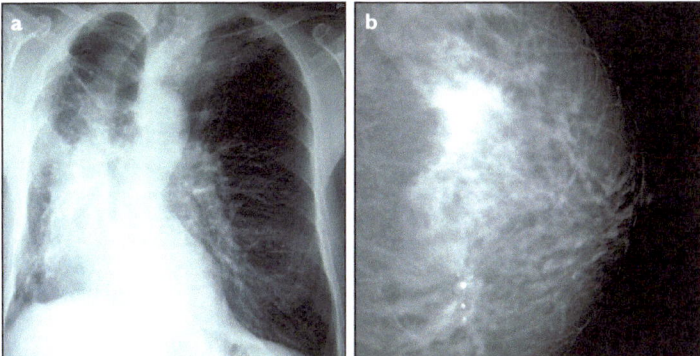

Fig. 8 a, b. The transition from being a patient to being a customer implies a transformation of semiotics: there are fewer and fewer gross lesions (**a**) and more indirect or minor indications (**b**)

Semiotics also – as described later – is no longer the same as in the past for the simple reason that the remarkable increase in sensibility of the various methods (that can be identified by diagnostic anticipations in the preclinical phase in screening programs) has changed the presentation of lesions. Lesions now no longer take the form of masses or neoformations – i.e., direct signs – but of convergences or distortions – i.e., indirect signs (Fig. 8).

So the problem is: are these rapid changes in imaging and semiotics supported by an equally rapid adaptation of the report – the method the radiologist uses to interpret and pass on new data to the prescribing physician? In other words, how is the report formulated today?

Chapter 2
From Images to the Technical and Ethical Responsibilities of Reporting

SEEING IS KNOWING

A description of the world in images is one of the elements that characterize the era of technical dominion. And yet, the myth of gaining knowledge through images – the idea that knowing is, before all else, being able make an image of something – is an ancient dream, and we might almost say, a necessary destiny. Indeed, Western culture has always been an essentially visual culture. The very word idea, which for Plato was the most appropriate object of knowledge, etymologically derives from *orao*, a very ancient verb that means to see.

To have an idea about something therefore implies having some image of it. Thanks to the image, the eye that looks at it can measure, can make a more exhaustive and detailed examination of the thing; it can compare and put items side by side in a series to discover similarities and diversities. In the contemplation, which is the closest point that the person looking and the object being looked at come together, the eye itself almost seems to disappear and become one with the image. When contemplating, the eye forgets its inclinations and interrupts its interests, obtaining a more objective and perfect vision, where the highest level of adaptation is noted between what is said and thought and things as they are. The radiologist, who looks and contemplates, also knows. Later, it will be necessary to capture the specificity of this act of seeing. We must never forget that the images used are the product of refined and extremely complicated technological processes whose action, which is not at all evident and natural, accompanies and conditions the specific act of looking, which is absolutely natural, that every radiologist carries out.

IMAGES AND WORDS

Viewing an image does not occur by chance, but according to a recurring scheme. It is the highest point of a certain process, which the ancients called dialectics. From a situation of initial obscurity, where nothing can be seen, we arrive at an idea, which is the most suitable image of the thing. This is reached by *dia-logos*, in other words, through (*dia*) speech (*logos*). The Greeks, therefore, already clearly understood the essential link between viewing an image and speech. The person contemplating not only arrived at the vision through dialogue, but then communicated the truth of what was seen in the dialogue. This nearness of image and speech has often led to concealment of their essential differences, leading us to believe in their possible identification.

We believe such misunderstanding lies in the idea whereby image and speech share a sign structure. The sign structure is essentially one of cross-reference. Image and speech do not speak for themselves, but each stands for the other. Generally, this can be interpreted in two ways:

1. The image is a kind of speech: in other words, each image behaves like the signs of a language. It not only depicts; it also speaks of the items it depicts.
2. Speech is a kind of image: it stands for the thing that is being spoken of, just as the image stands for the thing it depicts. In this way, the existence of the language is completely condensed to the relationship of depicting.

Perhaps the first thesis is true; pictographic writing has provided it, but if we think about this aspect carefully, it is not very interesting. Every object can be taken as a sign of something else, and therefore in general as a language. The problem is that a response like this leads to a loss of differences; there is a risk that we may neglect the image detail, if something like the image detail already exists.

On the other hand, the second thesis is sustainable, although it, too, encounters difficulties. To say that speech is image means to reduce all possibilities of the meaning of language to the depicting methods. Words, propositions, and the complex systems of signs that we use in order to be understood should create a kind of enormous mirror in which all the facts of the world are depicted. However, we all know that a dog depicted in a photograph of a dog is quite different from depicting a dog by using the word dog. Speech is in no way similar to the object, whereas the image is its perfect copy. Not only that. There is still the problem of the many different languages. If I say dog in English and cane in Italian, I evidently want to indicate the same object but I know that I am indicating the same object only if I know both the languages. In fact, if an Englishman and an Italian meet and neither knows the other's language, it would be quite difficult for them to know that dog and cane mean the same thing. In order to realize that, they would have to meet a dog or have the image of a dog. By reciprocally showing the real dog or its image to one another, and saying the words describing the animal in their respective languages, they would finally understand each other. This example may seem quite trivial, but it is not. It is proof that a real difference exists between an image and speech: whereas the former refers directly to what it depicts, so much so that it is immediately understood by all, the latter may lead to misunderstanding, because it is not univocal and often it is also subjective. Yet, we entrust the interpretation of images that we see to the words that come to our mouth, with the illusion that these words can act as simple substitutes of the same images, and therefore, are characterized by the immediacy and naturalism of the reference. Are we right in doing this? Is this good practice? I think it is worthwhile to ask ourselves these questions.

RADIOLOGISTS: MANUFACTURES OF WORLDS

We shall try to deal with the matter that has just been raised by describing the topic of cross-reference in greater detail. Images and words, we have said, refer to something else: they stand for objects and facts in the world. This is certainly true; however, it does not exhaustively include the whole truth, especially if we focus carefully on the structure of the image.

Now, what is an image? We said that an image is a kind of sign. When we say this, we do immediately not think of the image but of its significance – the fact that it refers to something else, to its reference, to the thing that is depicted, to the object. In other words, we forget the image and we immediately look in the direction of *for*, that is, what the image *stands* for. We forget that besides *for*, the image also *stands*. The image, before referring to something else, stands alone, on its own.

The image (and this is mainly true for the technical type of images we are dealing with), in turn, is a material object, a thing that has an inner structure that is not exhausted in the act of simply referring to something else. From this point of view, the image is first of all an object that stands for another object. It is made of a certain material and is produced according to a certain process, it can be transported and manipulated, and its representing capacity depends on some characteristics that make it more or less suited to the scope. An out-of-focus image, like an image that is too dark or too light, does not capture the subject. A CT scan enables greater diagnostic precision than does a traditional type of X-ray because it is also a different object; it is made and viewed differently. So here it is not only a matter of quantity but quality and therefore of characteristics that often cannot be compared. Of course, a phoneme and a grapheme also show some material consistency, but I doubt that the level of complication, inherent to the word dog, as a sound or a sign, can even be vaguely compared with the complex nature of the construction of any image of a dog. All this to say that the image deserves and must be made into the topic, not only by virtue of the fact that it is representative of something, but precisely because it is a specific and particular object – different from speech – and the radiologist acts accordingly.

The point is this: in the case of the image, there is not only the sign relation – a depiction, a description, a meaning – but the image itself becomes the thing that is represented, that is described, the meaning – in one word, the object. The image attaches so closely to the thing it depicts that it eventually replaces it. The image is no longer a sign of the reality but reality itself, and faced with the image, we behave as if it were reality itself. I would even say something more. We have the impression that for certain types of images, it is no longer possible to speak of true and false. And this is for the simple reason that the reality the images portray is not in front of us, close at hand, but is entirely constructed by the image itself. And this situation is different from being a copy of reality: our technological iconic production processes do not produce simple photographs; they produce reality. For this reason, we like to think of radiologists as manufacturers of worlds.

This emphasis of the fact that the image must be seen as an object in itself poses a problem. In this way, it is no longer a sign we can use to describe and interpret; it is the thing that has to be described and interpreted. The image, in its presence as an object, then becomes opaque and often has no meaning because it is too complicated and not easy to interpret. Our technological images are so elaborate that only the well-trained eye of the specialist with experience can understand them. Yet these are very detailed images, and for this reason, they should immediately refer to the reality, but this is not the case. Most people cannot understand them and therefore are unable to distinguish anything significant in them.

In this condition, then, we must find other signs that express the sense of the image. The problem is to understand whether this sense can be an imaginative type of sense. Or rather, can we use another image to give a sense to an image, to interpret it? We can; but in actuality, this almost never happens because an image can be the sign of another image only if it is depicted. An image can only become the image of another image, but to be the image of an image means being the same image. Therefore, we have made no progress in the comprehension of images because we remain in the field of images. We can produce millions of images of an image, and maybe we can even come up with new processing techniques, but our image is always there, waiting for someone to look at it and understand it.

Interpretation must therefore be a primarily linguistic fact. In other words, to interpret images, we need a common system of signs and meanings that is more extensive than that of the images. In order to interpret the images, we need words and the extraordinarily complex nature of the uses and combinations that words can give life to. So, comprehension of the image is always and only a linguistic comprehension. Words can never be rejected by the image.

> **Top Tip!**
> And consequently, our first conclusion:
> Reporting is not an extra element but a component and essential part of the process of viewing-comprehending-interpreting images.

SEEING IS NOT TALKING

Everything okay? No, unfortunately it is not. The fact is that in real terms, the passage from the image to the word is never that simple and immediate. This is due to any number of reasons. In the first place, this is because the image has a logic that is different from the logic of the word. In the second place, this is because the image often proposes such a complex construction of the object that perhaps there is no appropriate word for it. When faced with a technical image, not only may the lay person but at times even the physician find himself or herself literally speechless. Let us take a brief look at the two following cases, as often the image proposes a complex construct.

In the logic of the image in general, the prevailing thing is the continuous rather than the discreet. If from the image I remove one of its parts, one of its elements, not only will the image no longer have the same meaning, but often, it will no longer have any meaning at all. Not only that: once the removed element has been split from the original image it belonged to, it will become unusable at the level of sense. It will no longer make any sense. This does not occur for the written and spoken word. Single words can still be used, like pieces of phrases perhaps deprived of the single parts. To the contrary, it is in fact this possibility of fragmenting and dividing that allows the words to always recompose senses. This is not the case for images, which do not lend themselves to bricolage, except to a limited extent.

So the image is global and, we would venture, often total. The vision of the image is essentially affected by this fact. It never requires an analytic interpretation, done in pieces and according to a set order, such as when we read a written text or when we write. In the image, the first glance is at the whole. We take a global look, which is often decisive in order to comprehend the sense, and that then directs a series of successive glances of a localized nature – of subsequent accumulations of the attention that takes place without a specific order and not necessarily on the whole surface of the image.

This is a disseminated interpretation, by detail, now here, now there, that does not always lead to a uniform acquisition of information between the various moments or even to logical consequentiality. Interpretation of the image has no ordered direction and not even a logical-temporal continuity. The problem is to turn this discontinuity of the vision of the image into the continuity of the written and the spoken word. Here, syntax has its own direction, its own one-dimensionality, that of the sequence, and it is to this one-dimensionality itself that getting across the sense of the words is connected to.

We cannot talk the same way we look (at something), and the price of this is often loss of information that we wanted to get across. Let us look at some of the problems.

THE PROBLEMS OF SUMMING UP

Often, we conceive the linguistic interpretation of the image, the report, as a summary. The problem is that in the world of images, there is no such thing as a summary. People who live in a world of images or in worlds built of different types of image have a tough relationship with conceptual summary. Summarizing a text means transferring the same content with new words, perhaps by reducing their number. We make a summary of it, an operation that we have been used to doing since early childhood. But there is no such thing as a summary in the world of images. An image never summarizes another image; it represents it, as we have already seen. The image of an image is always the same image. Not only that, the summing up is not a simple mechanical, quantitative operation in which something is said with fewer words; it is the product of a reorganization of the sense that may result from the comprehension of a text. A poor summing up is often the symptom of a poor understanding. So, the problem is the following: how can we pass from the world of images, characterized by the discontinuity and the analytical part of the vision, to the world of conceptual summing up that is implemented in the written and spoken word?

This is no trifling question. A virtuoso of vision is not necessarily a good writer or speaker. To the contrary, in the passage from image to word, we often find problems. We cannot find the right words to express what we have seen. A lot of the effort that goes into reporting lies in this movement that is as complex as it is essential.

FROM THE TRUTH OF THE IMAGE TO THE SENSE OF THE WORDS

Here we spend a moment investigating the question of language. In the passage from the image to the word, a very important logical passage – which is often neglected – comes into play. We will attempt to retrace this with you beginning from the classic discussion conducted by G. Frege in an important paper written in 1892, called "Sense and Denotation".

We take the liberty of asking you a question: is there any difference between the expressions $a = a$ and $a = b$ where a and b indicate the same object? If there is a difference, what is it? If there is a difference between the two expressions, does this difference apply to the objects indicated by the letters a and b or only the signs a and b? Now, this difference cannot apply to the object, because we have assumed that the object is the same, so it must apply to the signs used. Let's as say that in both $a = a$ and $a = b$, an equal relationship between the signs is expressed.

Still, the two expressions are different: in the former, the sign a is placed on an equal footing with itself; in the second, the sign a is placed on an equal footing with b. The fact that we attribute a different cognitive value to the two expressions derives from this. In the former case, equality does not seem to add anything to our knowledge; in the latter case, it can be interesting to know that $a = b$. In sum, the second relationship of identity, $a = b$, seems to effectively expand our knowledge. Many of our scientific reports on the objects of knowledge (and of our problems regarding the language to use) often have their roots in the difficulty of setting up an equal relationship between the signs we use to indicate objects.

Let us observe the following expressions:
"The evening star = the morning star".

Here we have the same object (the planet Venus) that is named with two different senses. When we talk, we need to distinguish between the object we are talking about (for the logicians, denotation) and the sense we use to talk about it. We can talk about the same object in different senses, as in the example we just saw. This implies that the sense – in other words, the words of the report – is to a certain extent independent from the things, at least to the extent that given an object, all the ways it can be named are not predetermined a priori.

> **Top Tip!**
>
> The name is not the object. The report is not the image. The image of the object does not predetermine the language to describe it, a priori. So, the fact of establishing equality or agreement between two different names of an object can be translated into a successful communication. Otherwise, a misunderstanding will occur.

To say that the sense of an expression is independent from the object it expresses does not imply stating that the sense is something not objective. Above all, it does not imply that the sense is eminently subjective for that reason. The sense – in other words, the word – lies somewhere between the object in the image and the subjective representation we have. Let us imagine contemplating the planet Venus. Here we have an object (the planet), its subjective representation (the visual impression on the retina – maybe even accompanied by thoughts and emotions), and an expression (the evening star), which although not identified with the object cannot be reducible to the contingent and subjective elements of the situation, either.

The expression "the evening star" is, of course, partial, because it expresses a possible sense used to verbalize the object, Venus, but it is agreed by several interlocutors, and can be put into an equal or unequal relationship with other expressions. If the problem of the report is identified with the problem of the sense, we have to conclude that in the leap from image (object) to word, we do not have a passage between objective and subjective but between one type of objectivity and another type of objectivity: between the objectivity of the object itself and the objectivity of the word (which is not reduced to the former, because the word is not the image and because – if it were not thus – we would have resolved all these problems, and there would be no need for any book on reporting).

> **Top Tip!**
>
> Rather, the objectivity of the word has something to do with the linguistic agreement of the expressions used; in other words, with the fact that the sense is a public fact, possessed not by one but by many speakers.

We have comprehended that whereas the word is not objective in the sense that an image can be, neither is it subjective. Still, in the case of the report, to what extent can the sense of the words be independent from the image? Let us look at the following statement, which contains not only names or expressions indicating single objects, but also contains relations and predications relative to the objects. In general, we use these complex statements when we need to describe objects that have properties:

"Ulysses was disembarked at Ithaca while he was in a deep sleep".

Here we have a complex statement expressing the case of a given object "Ulysses", while he was in the state of "of deep sleep", who was subjected to the action of "being disembarked" on an island, called "Ithaca". Now, it is clear that we are talking about a statement that has an agreed sense, we understand this completely, a great poet wrote it, and perhaps we have even uttered it. Still, may I please ask you: what object does this statement refer to? What is its overall value of truth? What does it describe? In sum: what does it tell me about the world?

In trying to answer these questions, we suddenly come up against some really serious problems. This statement, although it has an objective sense, cannot truly and objectively refer to any situation because there is no way we can find an object of reference for the name Ulysses. We can go to Ithaca and perhaps if we wait patiently and observe, we may see someone being disembarked while sleeping, but it is highly unlikely that we will ever see Ulysses himself sleeping while he disembarks onto his island.

Here, the lack of objective reference of the statement does not allow the whole statement to have any truthful value as regards the situation described. The name Ulysses is, therefore, the same as the following nominal expression:

"The furthest planet from the Earth".

This expression undoubtedly makes sense. Indeed, we could find it in some astronomy manual, but what does it denote? To what object does it refer? In what region of reality do we need to look to find such an object? In fact, it is doubtful that an object of this kind exists. This expression, although comprehensible and although so similar to a scientific proposition, appears completely indeterminate as regards the object it is supposed to denote. This is why it is hard for it to be accepted in a serious scientific report on what is or is not in the universe. This leads to the formulation of a significant restriction as regards linguistic expression in reporting:

> **Top Tip!**
> When a report is written, it is not only intended to offer thoughts that can be agreed upon and reasonable, but also to express statements that have the value of truth on taking up or not taking up a given situation.

In order for this to occur – in other words, for the report to really be informative about a given situation, or in other words, until it has been given the value of truth – two conditions must be met:
1. That every expression of the report given in the form of a name or of a nominal expression in fact denotes an object.
2. That no new sign or group of signs is introduced as a name without this being guaranteed a specific meaning.

Every ambiguity regarding the meaning of the signs indicating objects is reflected in an ambiguity on the overall value of truth of the situation described. These conditions allow us to formulate a real standard logical principle for reporting that could sound like this:

> **Top Tip!**
> In reporting, the meaning of a complex expression depends on the meaning of its parts.

In the passage from image to word, we express a sense: the sense of the image. This sense has its own objectivity, which is different and autonomous from that of the image. An image can be reported in different senses, even if all those senses refer to the same image. This diversity is seen as a positive resource; the freedom of the radiologists, their technical knowledge, and their linguistic skills are expressed in this. They can look for the most widely accepted and most informative sense for colleagues and patients, because the sense is possessed by many and not by one.

Still, this autonomy of the sense of the words depicting the image is also a danger. If I say:

"The present king of France is bald."

Of course, it expresses something that means something but that is unfortunately false. No object X is given to prove that X is king of France and that said X is bald. Now, the sense can mask the falseness and take the reader off the track of the purpose. Still, the same proposition also gives some indications to control its truth. The word present indicates to us the area of reality within which we must search for the object. It is the present time, and in this area of reality, it is easy to see that no king of France exists, even less so one without hair. This reminds us that apart from the sense in the report, we believe we always need to have in our sights what we would call the "overall value of truth" of the expressions used – in other words, the informative effectiveness on what exists and what does not exist in the world at the present time. For this to happen, we must avoid any ambiguity in the meaning of the nominal terms used (nouns, technical names, participles), because every vagueness of the parts can lead to a vagueness in the meaning of the whole.

WRITING

We must not forget another aspect. In the report, the meaning is not expressed orally but in writing. This generates additional difficulties and dangers. As far as writing is concerned, we must always consider the following elements:
1. Writing helps the memory but it also freezes it.
2. Writing takes the report away from its author and allows it to be interpreted in his/her absence.
3. After being written, the report can no longer be defended and explained by its author.

4. Writing cannot be made clearer or more complete; what is written is written!

Writing is indispensable; it establishes the meaning of the report and allows it to be transmitted, but it can also betray it. A written text can be interpreted in various ways and in the absence of the author. This may be fine for a literary text, but it is not so desirable for a report. The report is an indispensable tool for treatment; it soothes and heals, but it must be written accurately, otherwise it may poison and kill. Ever since the dawn of our civilization, the word *farmacon* has existed, which exactly expresses the dual condition to which the report is subjected. *Farmacon*, in fact, means both medicine and poison. The same applies to the report: it is a treatment, the beginning of every other treatment, but it can fail and become poison if it does not achieve its objective, which is the effective transmission of a shared meaning.

> **Top Tip!**
> In a nutshell, a report is like a drug. The report is the radiologist's drug.

REPORTING AND RESPONSIBILITY

When looking at an image, we often simply linguistically repeat – using phonemes and graphemes – the image itself. That is, we describe it. But a description does not add anything to an image. Words are not only used to describe but have other, infinite, uses. We do many different things with words. Furthermore, each act of communication, both verbal and written, even the most neutral and objective description, is aimed at someone.

This someone is not always the same someone. Consequently, in order to arrive effectively, our act of communication must come to grips with the specific otherness of the person it is aimed at. In Western tradition, the interpreter, the reader of signs and images, is a mediator. In this mediation, not only does the interpreter insert the entire self – inclinations and interests – but also turns to other people – to their interests, to their inclinations, and to their lives. The interpreter has a tremendous destiny – the spokesperson of the gods, of their sometimes dramatic and unacceptable messages. But he or she must pluck up courage, know how to speak well, and realize that not only is there an ethics of communication but that communication itself is configured as ethics.

The current discussion, not only at the philosophical level but also more specifically aimed at the definition of a standard of judgment as regards professional conduct, has identified the concept of responsibility as the decisive word around which our reflection must pivot. The definition of responsibility as an ethical inclination to determine or correct our behavior on the basis of the possibility of knowing its effects in advance is mainly based on the understanding of the activity of humans according to the category of power. We are only responsible if we have the power to act in such a way as to determine real consequences for ourselves and for other people. The total incapacity of producing effects, physical or intellectual as they may be, cannot be considered as responsibility. This means that a physically immobile individual, though perfectly healthy from the mental point of view, would be able to conceive actions to be performed by other people. The individual could have someone killed or could give bad advice, generating negative consequences for that individual and for others. If this happened, such an individual would not only be just as responsible as the people who acted but even more so because the individual was the source of every consequent negative effect. The power of acting intellectually is no less than the power of acting physically.

This explains the attention that law has always paid to the juridical position of the instigator and the extreme harshness of the sentences handed out for crimes such as conspiracy, even if they produced no appreciable effects. Those who plan a terrorist deed but do not have the time to carry it out commit a very serious crime, regardless of the consequences it could have had. The power of acting, therefore, means not the effective performance of an action but the capacity to prepare it in all its consequences.

> **Top Tip!**
> The power of doing that has effects on other people is the horizon of responsibility.

The sphere of reporting is fully incorporated in that of responsibility. In it, the power of doing is connected with writing. The report is not just an expression of theoretical competence but is also a concrete action – a drug, as we said before. The information contained in the report generates effects that have consequences to other people.

Of course, this not only involves the specific activity of radiologists but also that of doctors in general. Now, what does being responsible mean for the doctor at a purely philosophical level? First of all, it means that his or her actions are seen as a capacity of doing, as a power, therefore. The doctor wanted this power, or at least one hopes so. The doctor became a doctor by deliberately studying medicine and then deciding to sit for competition exams or obtain qualifications to enter the profession. There was no obligation to do so; the intent was to try to do something for somebody else. By doing so, the doctor becomes responsible. However, it is not only the initial choice of becoming the cause of effects for other people that makes the doctor responsible, but also the excess of power the doctor wields. The doctor knows more about medicine than do other people, both in terms of quantity and quality. Moreover, that knowledge is seen as a power, not only because it is greater, but also because it concerns what is of great interest to other people: health – organic integrity – without which no other integrity is possible. What the doctor implements with action interests the other person, not in an occasional or superficial way, but as regards what that other person is and desires to be.

The doctor's position in the action circuit is typically that of a moral agent. We should point out that in this context, moral does not mean good or bad, and not even something that has something to do with emotions or pity. On the contrary, being a moral agent is something very technical, which concerns the specific position occupied in the relationship with other people. More precisely, being a moral agent expresses the specific position of someone who occupies the starting position in a chain of effects and consequences. If I let someone get into my car and I start driving, I am responsible in two ways: (a) I deliberately chose to drive; (b) the other person cannot drive and therefore I have more power than that person does. However, how far does this power go? It is limited and governed by the other person's life. This applies both whether I decide to drive too fast or whether I drive prudently. As long as I am driving, for as long as I exercise a power on the existence of another person, I am responsible for that person. This is why we must drive with skill and competence. My power of doing makes me responsible, which means that I must do everything I can to avoid an accident or a harmful effect on the person who has submitted to my action.

This example reveals a further aspect, the power of doing, which for the radiologist is the knowledge-power of writing, which makes one responsible; however, not unlimitedly responsible. The same power that confers responsibility also limits it. In fact, no one can be blamed for damage that he or she was unable to cause or avoid. If the radiologist uses his or her skills and capacities to a maximum but, despite, the patient cannot be saved, the radiologist cannot be held responsible for the negative outcome that was determined starting from the report. Those who know can, and those who can are responsible for their power, but only as regards what is within their power.

This discussion allows us to draw an important conclusion: if the power of writing is the extent of the responsibility of the radiologist, and he or she is more responsible the more he or she knows how to use this power, this means that the radiologist must want to exercise this power as effectively as possible. In other words, the technique of reporting must not be subject to limitations as regards its capacity of acting as a drug. It must be constantly developed and strengthened as regards its specific possibilities. Whereas it is true that power increases responsibility, it is also true that it always establishes a new definition, up to the point that a technically less powerful reporting technique can generate much greater damage, and be morally censured, than a more updated and effective reporting method.

Top Tip!

The report expresses the radiologist's power of doing and, therefore, the extent of his or her responsibility. However, this power must not be limited but strengthened in all its possibilities. Only in this way can it fully satisfy the requirement to produce not damage, but the maximum amount of positive consequences and well-being for other people.

Chapter 3
Medical-Legal Aspects

A good definition of a report that can be used for this chapter is: "The report is the subjective interpretation of objective data by a professional".

There are several medical-legal aspects to a report. First of all, as a written document, the report has the characteristics of a certificate, though it is not one. Like a certificate, it must be truthful; it must be a product of certainty – having an intrinsic legal value. Therefore, equally, the report is a declaration of science aimed at the same use as the certificate, also taking on the meaning of consultation, as it is a "motivated opinion" to the request of a colleague.

From this point of view, the requirements of the report are of twofold: (a) substantial (truthfulness; completeness; precision; clarity; and especially, contextualization, that is, the exact attribution to the person); (b) formal, which also becomes substantial (place of issue; date and, eventually, time of the exam, which can be very important in emergencies; and the doctor's first name, surname, full signature, and function).

With the report, the radiologist must produce a document that certifies the truth, just like a certificate. Therefore, assumptions of falsity in a public document in the report, over and above the medical evaluation, can be made as regards date, site, name, anatomical region, etc. In other words, when the report incorrectly marks the site of the exam or the anatomical region, the truth has not been told, and therefore the formal and substantial concept of the certificate has been breached (Fig. 9).

[...] Lumbar magnetic resonance (MR) examination identified as dorsal MR: this is false (ideological) because it does not correspond to the facts.

Fig. 9. Report error that can be defined as "false ideological"

Another assumption is the following: the report is the final product of the radiologist's activity, not toward the patient but toward the person. That is, not the patient in the generic sense of the word, but the human being, who can suffer mental, moral, material, or physical consequences due to the report.

Another very important point is that the report layout must be very strict. There must be a strict parallelism between its parts (clinical information, method of execution, description, conclusions, and eventual continuation of exams), and it must truly reflect the role it plays in the clinical and anamnestic sphere of that patient (initial exam, eventually in the form of a structured report; follow-up exam; or additional exam) (Fig. 10). All these are distinctions – the first and the second – that we will talk about more specifically in other chapters. All this goes beyond the guidelines, where existing, or personal habits and national tendencies, because in the end, the report – apart from its diagnostic and communicative qualities – must respect the story of the patient and the professionalism of the other doctors, both those who are radiologists and those who are not.

We can compare the compilation of a report with that of a school essay, the title of which is none other than the clinical information or diagnostic suspect, that is, the "motivated request". The subject – the report – is written so as to show a balance between its parts and the title; that is, between the interpretation and the diagnostic suspect. Therefore, the technical methods of execution – if the requested exam implies a choice in this sense – is the first phrase of the essay, indicating the method used to write it, immediately demonstrating that one has tried to understand the title – that is, the meaning of the request – and thus playing the role of the clinical radiologist (Fig. 11). The description of the semiological elements is the largest part of the essay. Therefore, it should not be too long, as it would become prolix, nor too short, as it would be superficial. It should be commensurate to the title of the essay. The diagnostic conclusion should be the nodal point, a consequence of the previous sections. Given

a

The test is carried out because of epigastralgia and weight loss.
[...] At the head of the pancreas, there is a solid hypoechogenic lesion, with a diameter of about 2 cm, which does not have clearly marked borders. There is a dilatation of the biliary tracts, both intra- and extrahepatic. [...] Conclusions: suspected pancreatic heteroplasia. It is necessary to follow this up with computed tomography.

b

The test is carried out to integrate the previous echography of ..., first with a multilayer technique, and then with a means of contrast with acquisition during the arterial, portal, and late phases.
The expansive cephalopancreatic lesion is confirmed, with a maximum diameter of 2 cm ...
The lesion does not infiltrate the upper mesenteric vein and arteries. There are no lymphadenomegalies or focal hepatic lesions.

c

Control following a duodeno-cephalo-pancreasectomy.
Compared with the previous computed tomography of the abdomen dated..., results of the resection of the known cephalopancreatic lesion are visible. There are no sign of relapse of the illness in the affected area. As far as the rest is concerned, the picture is unchanged, in particular, there are no hepatic foci lesions or lymphadenomegalies.

Fig. 10 a-c. Typical examples of **a** structured report in the first examination (echography of the abdomen), **b** integrating examination (computed tomography of the abdomen), and **c** check examination (computed tomography of the abdomen)

the semiological elements described, and in the wake of the chosen methodology, the most probable diagnostic hypothesis is the one formulated. For this reason, a "dry" diagnostic conclusion is not generally suitable, because – as will be discussed at a later stage – the radiologist is not conclusive but contributes, though in an often determining way, to the diagnostic "puzzle". But a conclusion with more than two hypotheses is also not appreciated, as it demonstrates to the prescriber that the radiologist has not fully understood the clinical request. Thus, it generates uncertainty and mistrust toward the radiologist, especially if that radiologist is reputed to be inconclusive and/or to ask for diagnostic completions too often (Fig. 12). Therefore, suggesting additional exams must demonstrate the radiologist's desire to draw a conclusion using common sense and determination but not imply professional insufficiency or inadequacy (Fig. 13).

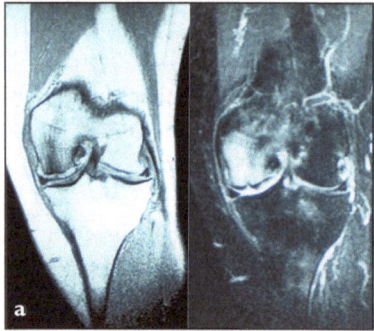
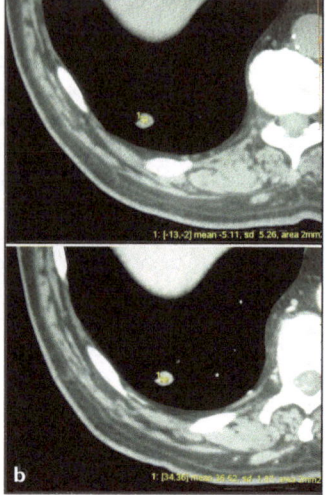

c
This test was requested due to a posttraumatic gonalgia, carried out utilizing T1- and T2-weighted sequences and fat suppression.
[...] There is an area of altered signal of the spongiosa ossea of the medial femoral condyle, characterized by gradient echo T1 hypointensity and SPIR T2 hyperintensity, compatible with edema-hyperemia. [...]
The clinical picture suggests a bone contusion.

d
This test is carried out before and after administering, if necessary, a contrast medium, with a protocol for the study of the characterization of the nodular lesion.
[...] The nodule presents an increase in density after administering contrast equal to about 40 Hounsfield units. [...]
The clinical picture does not allow us to exclude the possible proliferative nature of the lesion, and resection in video-assisted thoracic surgery is recommended.

Fig. 11 a-d. Report understood as the harmonic development of a heading ("motivated request").
- Technical modalities of execution: **a** Spin echo and spectral presaturation inversion recovery magnetic resonance (MR) sequences of the knee requested for contusive trauma. **b** Pulmonary computed tomography (CT) scan without and with contrast medium to identify the density difference of a pulmonary nodule to be typified
- Description of semiological elements: **c** Medical report of the MR of the knee due to traumatic contusion. **d** Medical report of the CT of the lungs

a *In the eighth segment of the liver, there is a solid hyperechogenic solid for-mation, with a diameter of about 3 cm. compatible with a first hypothe-sis, with an angioma, but which requires clinical analysis and a further analysis carried out through computed tomography. [...]*

b *[...] Solid formation, homogeneously hypodense at the first examination, and hyperdense after administering contrast agent, compatible with an ini-tial hypothesis of angioma. In order to be able to formulate a more reli-able evaluation, it is opportune to carry out further analysis with a magnetic resonance test.*

c *This test confirms the result of the computerized tomography of a ho-mogeneously hyperintense formation in the T2-weighted sequences, char-acterized – after gadolinium contrast agent – by a progressive centripetal impregnation, which appears to be almost complete at a later stage. These results are compatible with a hepatic angioma. [...]*
Echographic controls over time are recommended.

Fig. 12 a-c. Inconclusive medical reports (**a**, echography; **b**, computed tomography), with the indication of carrying out further tests (**c**, magnetic resonance), generating, therefore, uncertainty and lack of confidence in the doctor who prescribed them, es-pecially as the recommendations come from the same radiologist

a *[...] Stenosis of the proximal tract of the internal right carotid can be quantified between 60% and 80% of the vascular lumen. [...] A magnetic resonance angiography is recommended.*

b *[...] The stenosis identified affects the initial tract of the internal right carotid artery and does not seem to be of significance. In particular, it does not seem to exceed the 50–60% of the vascular width. [...]*
An echographic color-Doppler of the internal right carotid artery, carried out after an appropriate period of time, is recommended.

Fig. 13 a, b. Professional inadequacy may be expressed with the suggestion that fur-ther examinations be done. **a** After recommendation that the echographic color-Doppler of the supraaortic trunks be augmented with an magnetic resonance angiography (MRA), **b** the same radiologist advises that a further echographic color-Doppler be done to supplement the MRA

> **Top Tip!**
>
> In a nutshell, a tidy and balanced report, respectful of the clinical-anamnestic sequence, and clear and comprehensible, is the best medical-legal safeguard.

Let us take a look at other aspects. The report supposes that a diagnostic request has been made by the doctor in charge. That is, the motivated request is for an evaluation of the morbid process of his patient by the radiological specialist. The clinical request will be discussed more specifically later.

The report must comprise a complete and exemplary iconographic documentation, and it is indispensable to the doctor in charge when formulating a correct diagnosis combined with clinical and laboratory data. So, here is an open question: what role must the report play in the diagnosis; does it identify with it, or is it just a part of it, though essential? This affects the report's layout and, especially, its conclusion. In fact – as will be specified later – the diagnosis cannot be totally referred to the responsibility of the specialist doctor. It must be conceived as a puzzle comprising numerous harmoniously integrated pieces – the radiological exam being an important piece – that will be put together by the doctor in charge who, among other things, wants to put it together without being conditioned by a peremptory diagnosis made by the radiologist.

There are certainly radiological, ultrasound, tomodensitometric, and other images that are unequivocal and therefore pathognomonic for certain illnesses or injuries (Fig. 14). Equally, though, due to the complexity of biological phenomena, the question asked by the doctor in charge cannot always be immediately and completely answered; that is, the images can be deceiving and lead doctors to neglect or undervalue the clinical and anamnestic data (Fig. 15). The conclusion of a report should therefore be open to more than one diagnostic interpretation (not too many! as mentioned above), eventually with some differential diagnostic elements, in order to allow the doctor in charge to "manage" the procedure to the best, particularly in light of the other clinical-instrumental reports. If the exam has been requested as an integration of other ones, though, it has to be conclusive.

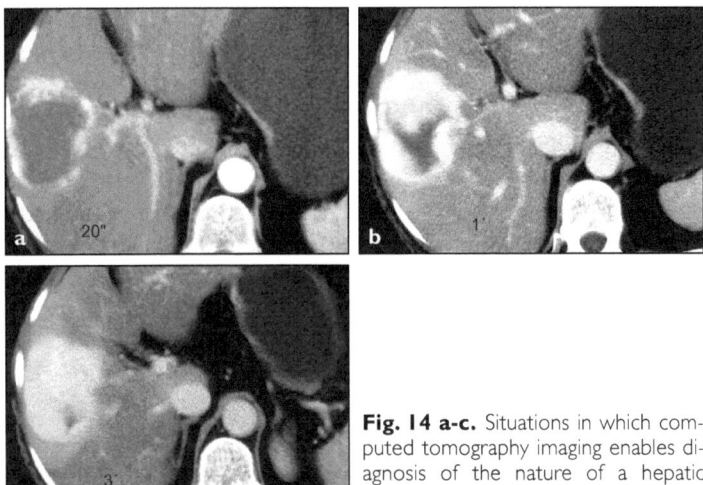

Fig. 14 a-c. Situations in which computed tomography imaging enables diagnosis of the nature of a hepatic hemangioma

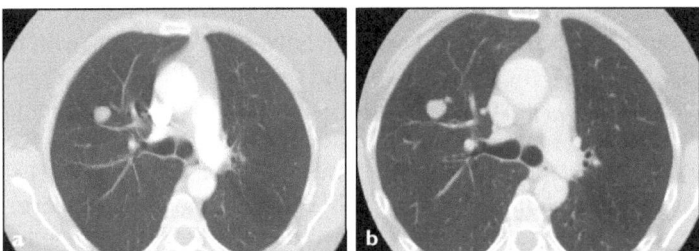

Fig. 15 a, b. Situations in which imaging is misleading and may lead to incorrect diagnosis of the nature of a lesion. **a** Solid formation in the right lung, interpreted as benign in computed tomography (CT) without and with contrast medium due to the limited enhancement. **b** Wrongly considered as unchanged when the check test was done 6 months later. The patient nevertheless chose to undergo surgical intervention rather than to continue with the checks: it was a case of adenocarcinoma

The report, therefore, is none other than the opinion of a professional, the only person qualified to give it and make it official in writing. In this sense, it only acts as proof toward the image that the radiologist decided to register and attach. Therefore, the conclusions of the report express the personal interpretation of that radiologist – which may be more or less shared by colleagues – and outline his or her personality and psychology; that is, the inclination to "compromise" himself or herself on the basis of the images produced (see chapter titled "The Psychology of a Good Report: Radiologist and User").

Some points should be made at this stage. The report must be clearly and legibly signed by the radiologist who drew it up, who – by doing so – accepts responsibility; or it must be initialed if the radiologist's name and surname are printed by computer (digital signature). The image must ensure precise and certain patient identification so there are no doubts as to the attribution of the exam ("falsity in a public document"; see above). It is an aspect that is not sufficiently evaluated by the radiologist, fortunately now made obsolete by radiology information system (RIS)/PACS integration.

The report must contain a technical description, not only for greater efficiency and completeness of interpretation – as mentioned above – but also for protection aspects, so as to enter the exposure dosage in the patient's health record. A very deeply felt forensic aspect in Italy is the obligation to store and archive such information. This is now discussed briefly. The subject is governed by Italian Legislative Decree 230/95, which, in article 114, includes among the responsibilities of the specialist that of "ensuring that the examinations and treatments with ionizing radiation are individually recorded". This decree would be incomplete on its own, but it was then partly repealed and completed by subsequent Legislative Decree 187/2000. The idea behind the two decrees is that that the local health districts must provide citizens with a free "personal radiological record" in which the competent specialist doctors must enter every exam involving the emission of X-rays according to methods that still remain to be defined. For example, the relationship between the radiological record and the all-inclusive personal health record that should have been given to every citizen as early as 1978, according to the law establishing the National Health Service; or operative limitation on specialists established in Legislative Decree 230/95, but not on the medical categories who exercise complementary radio diagnostics, such as dentists, or still, the information contained in the record, that is, if it must be limited to the dose – radiated or absorbed – or also extended to the report because, of course, its connotations would be very different. However, the legislators' idea is that the personal radiological record should be a "traveling" archive, updated by those providing the service and held and kept by the patient or the patient's legal representative.

But the stable recording and archiving of data is the responsibility of the doctor who produced the reports and images. This data must be stored in the health areas in which it is collected, according to the methods established in article 114 of Legislative Decree 230/95 and repeated in article 111 of the same decree and in the subsequent Ministerial Decree of 14 February 1997. This data must be available for at least 10 years for image documentation and without limits for reports drawn by specialists. Data can also be recorded on electronic supports. The law governing the method of recording and archiving digital reports is mentioned in the chapter titled "Structured Reports and PACS".

Returning to the report: Some points should be made concerning the language to use, the methods of its delivery to the patient or user, and the limits to the explanations that can be given to the patient, seeing that – as explained below – the patient is not the recipient of the report. As regards the first point – language – we must first decide who the report is written for, whether for the doctor in charge or for the patient. As the report is simply a consultation between two colleagues – the one who makes the request (motivated request) and the one who expresses the interpretation thanks to the technology used – it must be perfectly clear and intelligible to the doctor in charge. At the end of the day, it is this doctor for whom the report is written, and no objections can be made if it is incomprehensible to the patient. Therefore, the vocabulary must be technical-scientific and refer to the methods of execution (MR sequences; type and quantity of contrast agent, etc.), normal and pathological anatomy, physiopathology, radiological semiotics, and, especially, to the clinical picture. Ultimately, the more the report communicates effectively – that is, the clearer and more unequivocal it is, bearing in mind that the interlocutor is the prescriber – the less likely it is for there to be misunderstandings, "noise", between the radiologist and the doctor in charge.

Also, due to this requirement for clarity, the report – as will be explained later – is always the expression of the personality of the radiologist; that is, of his or her culture, experience, and clinical intuition. The need for clarity, however, does not justify reports that are so concise and synthetic as to be insufficient and superficial (Fig. 16). Because if, on the one hand, the increasingly more frenetic working rhythms, the eventual shortage of computer equipment, the overabundance of negative exams, and requests for medical-legal coverage only, invite radiologists to keep their reports essential, on the other hand, all this cannot justify laziness, which can perhaps be simulated by synthetic and/or memorized phrases. Neither

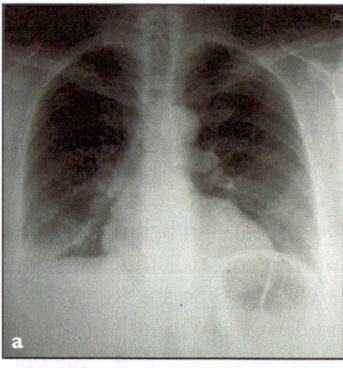
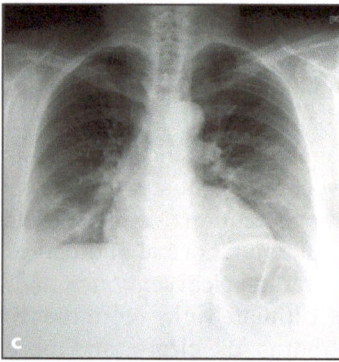

b
Pulmonary infiltration at the bottom right.

d
Control of the pneumonia foci noted on 28/09/06.
At the moment, the parenchymal infiltration indicated on the bottom right of the lung has partially regressed; it is associated with mild pleural effusion on the same side.
The remaining medical reports are unchanged: in particular, there are no further parenchymal lesions or foci evident; pulmonary hila and heart are within the limits of normality.

Fig. 16 a-d. Totally insufficient report (**b**) of a radiological exam of the thorax (**a**) carried out at the casualty department. It is later rectified (**d**) by the control test (**c**) without any inappropriate behavior toward the colleague. **b** In the first medical report, there is the indication of pulmonary infiltration only, without a description of its characteristics or elements of normality. **d** In the second medical report, the description is completed by the addition of the missing elements

must it be an alibi for underrating incidental reports, which today have no clinical importance but may be potentially useful in the future, such as anatomical variants (cervical rib, *pectus excavatum*, transitional vertebra, septum pellucidum), the results of previous fractures (ribs, vertebra, or long bones), or of other pathologies (specific, pleuritic, or cerebral ischemic-infarct results) (Fig. 17). The other two points, method of delivery and explanations, are more simple and limited.

Regarding the first point: Report delivery is now governed by Italian Legislative Decree 196/2003, completing Law 675,

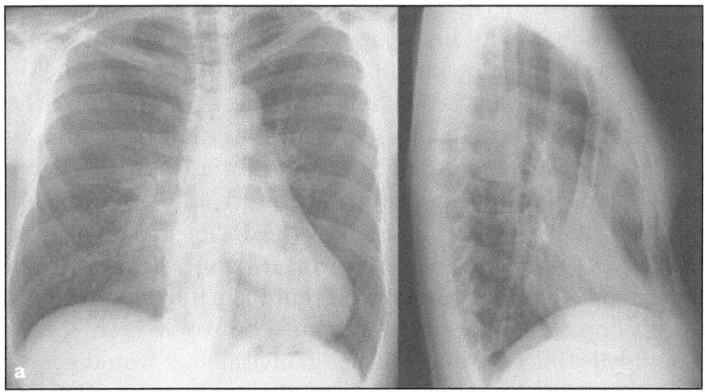
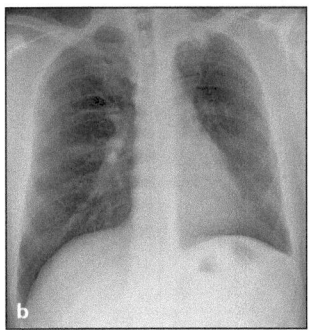
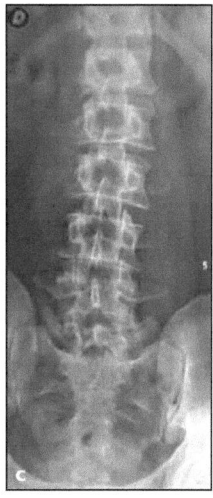

Fig. 17 a-c. Incidental medical reports, without a particular clinical significance, which are, however, to be included in the medical report, as they could be useful in following tests. **a** Pectus excavatum. **b** Results of previous tuberculosis on the left and of rib fractures on the right. **c** Transitional vertebra

better known as the privacy act. As the report contains the patient's personal data, it is always delivered in a closed envelope, clearly indicating that it contains confidential information and, as such, only accessible to the interested party or – following that party's express permission – to the doctor in charge.

Regarding the second point: if asked for explanations or clarifications by the interested party, that is, the patient or user, the radiologist can and must provide them, providing it is done in total respect of the ethical rules governing the relationship between the radiologist and the doctor in charge; that is, bearing in mind the work and professionalism of the other specialists. Furthermore, the patient exercises the power of self-determination of his or her state of health, for which reason he or she must be informed – the more so if he or she requests it – as to his or her real conditions. This allows the patient to authorize or refuse any further diagnostic investigations or determine therapeutic procedures (the well-known principle of informed consent). Therefore, any "convenient" reporting that may be requested by the doctor in charge or by the patient's family, such as *"ad usum delphini"* (AUD) or "copy for patient" (CFP), in order to prevent the patient from knowing his or her true state of health, must be avoided at all costs. Not only is this type of reporting inadvisable, it would generate several problems for the radiologist.

Chapter 4
Review of the Literature on Reports

Literature abounds in work on the report; in general, it gives guidelines or suggestions on communication efficiency. The literature agrees that the report is the only means of measuring the diagnostic ability – and, therefore, the professionalism – of the radiologist. It suggests which terms or expressions to use and which to avoid. It dictates which grammatical and lexical rules to respect. It discusses the main medical-legal aspects. It outlines the new technological scenarios – PACS and hospital information system (HIS)/RIS – that affect the way the reports are drawn up. It refers to the characteristics of modern imaging – panning and totipotent – to translate into the report. In other words, the pragmatic and efficient aspects of the report – certainly inviolable – are always taken into consideration.

The others – which in our opinion are even more inviolable because they necessarily precede the pragmatic and efficient aspects and qualify the radiologist as a specialist – are hardly considered in the literature at all. These are the human and humanistic aspects of the creation of the report and of the radiologist's comprehension of its importance for the patient/user (the power of the radiologist; see below), the ethical aspect of respect for the work of other professionals, and the logical-anamnestic aspect of the introduction of the report into a precise point in the patient's clinical history.

It is almost as if, in the logical construction of a path, some preliminary and/or collateral passages were left out, thus making the outcome incomprehensible or, at least, not very clear.

As a result, it is never emphasized that while the report is the subjective product of the professional who signs it and is responsible for it, it is also the outcome of the work of a team. That team comprises the patient, the doctor in charge, any other professionals involved, and previous or subsequent radiologists – each with precise tasks that, if not performed, would lower the quality of the report.

We propose to analyze all these aspects and "players" in the subsequent chapters.

Chapter 5
Current Health Needs

The main characteristics of industrialized societies are: as concerns demographics, a drop in birth rates, ageing of the native population, and immigration from poor countries; as concerns health, development and implementation of screening programs and – more generally speaking – preclinical diagnoses. These peculiar demographic and health aspects deeply affect reporting, as they outline (a) the prevailing type of population, and (b) emerging health needs. It is well known – as regards clinical radiology – that the report must interpret both as well as possible. Here, we take a closer look at them and explain how they affect reporting.

In an ageing population, there is a prevalence of chronic degenerative and invalidating pathologies, such as osteoarticular diseases in polyarthrosis sufferers and vertebral diseases in osteoporosis patients; cognitive pathologies, such as dementia; and motor pathologies, such as extrapyramidal diseases (Fig. 18). This means that, generally speaking, diagnostic exams will be requested in order to check whether known pathologies have stabilized or whether they have become acute. In other words, put extremely synthetically, where the population is elderly, "-osis" (degenerative) pathologies prevail, and exams are required in order to exclude "-itis" (acute) (Fig. 19). This allows us to deduce that two general aspects prevail: (a) the so-called follow-ups of previous exams of the same type within a reasonable period of time (especially the chest, the backbone, and osteoarticular sections), and (b) negativity reports, generally performed on healthy or presumably healthy people.

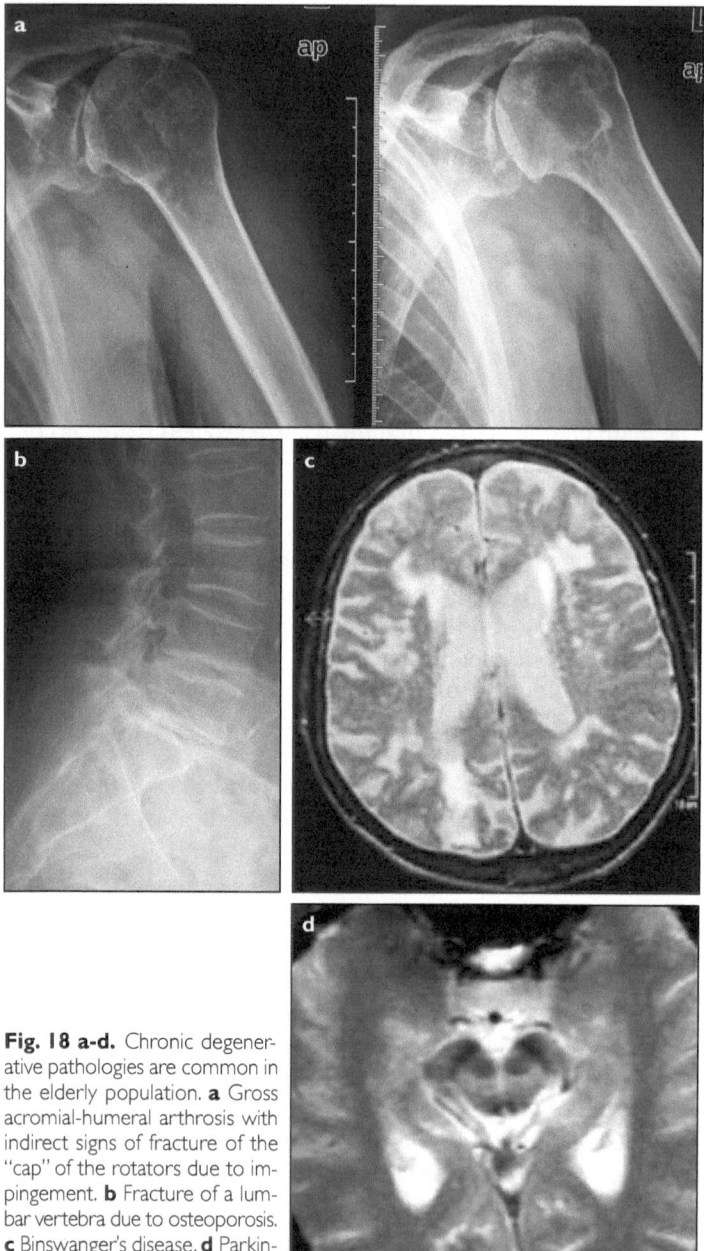

Fig. 18 a-d. Chronic degenerative pathologies are common in the elderly population. **a** Gross acromial-humeral arthrosis with indirect signs of fracture of the "cap" of the rotators due to impingement. **b** Fracture of a lumbar vertebra due to osteoporosis. **c** Binswanger's disease. **d** Parkinson's disease

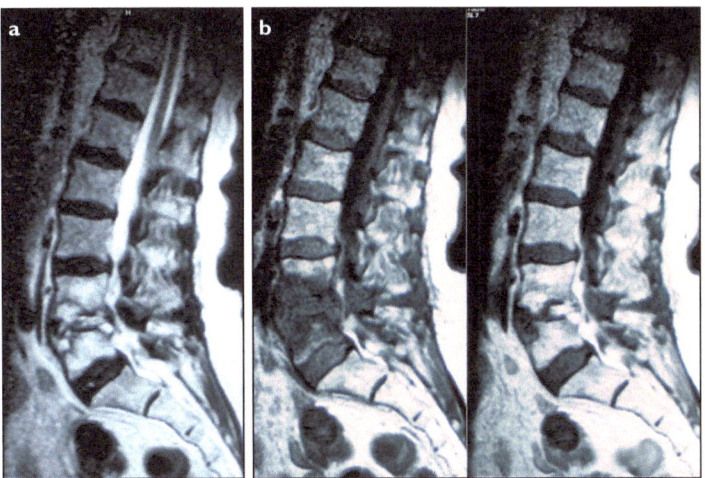

Fig. 19 a, b. Spondylodiscitis in an aged patient: **a** T2-weighted sagittal spin echo (SE) sequence. **b** T1-weighted sagittal SE sequences before and after injection of gadolinium

As regards point a: The content of the report must be specific; that is, it must mention the differences with respect to the previous exams or confirm the essential points of the stabilized radiological situation. This is because the prescriber of the exam may not be aware of the patient's radiological history, which, instead, the specialist knows thanks to the RIS (Fig. 20).

As regards point b: The target of normality for that type of exam is probably identified and must then be described. Also, the prescriber wishes to be reassured regarding the accuracy

Comparing it to the previous test of ... the appearance of a central posterior hernia of the disc L5–S1 with an impression/mark on the dural sac. The remaining results remain unchanged: in particular, a little intraforaminal hernia on the right of the disc L4–L5 is confirmed, with a compression on the spinal root.

Fig. 20. Magnetic resonance of the lumbar column; check examination. In the medical report about the control test, changes in the known medical picture are pointed out, and only the main unchanged aspects are stressed

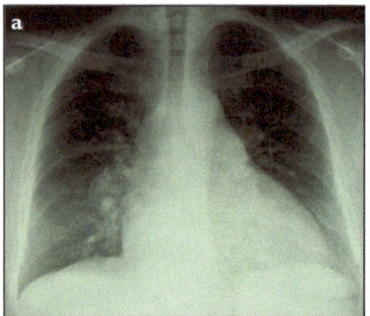

No actual focal pleuroparenchy-matous lesions. Heart image en-larged.

Fig. 21 a, b. Insufficient thorax radiogram report (**b**) in which the examination's qualifying elements are not all specified. In this case, the signs of the initial small circle's overload can be seen but are not described

of the radiologist's analysis (for example, normality of the thoracic X-ray or where it is complex and concerns several organs) (Fig. 21). On the other hand – in the event of a positive result – the radiological semiotic modifications, from patient to user, must be considered, as indicated in the "Introduction."

These aspects will be discussed in greater detail in the chapters "Principal Report Typologies" and "Radiological Semiotics in the Report". The relationship between current health needs and the consequent diagnostic exams is schematized in Table 1.

Table 1. Exhisting Sanitary Needs and Diagnostic Tests

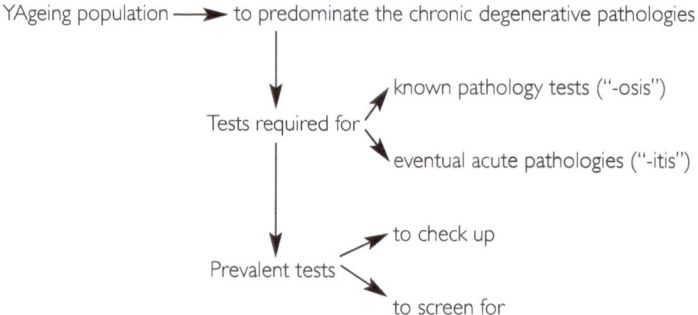

Chapter 6
Principal Report Typologies

The layout of the report cannot always be the same, because – as we have just pointed out – it depends on personal (RIS) and clinical data variables. Reports can therefore be grouped according to the following exam types:

1. Initial exam
2. Follow-up exam
3. Additional exam
4. Preventive exam

INITIAL EXAM

The patient is not known to the RIS of that service or has never been given the type of exam in question. For example, an extemporary or occasional first-aid service or a thoracic X-ray on a young person with no previous case history.

In this case, the report is drawn up in the conventional way for the type of exam in question: concise for a first-aid service (Fig. 22a); more articulated for other requests commensurate with their complexity, from the banal conventional osteoarticular exam (Fig. 22b) to MR or PET-CT-integrated imaging (Fig. 22c). Generally speaking, international literature only considers reports of this type, as though they were the only ones, and totally neglects all the others indicated below.

COMPARATIVE OR FOLLOW-UP EXAM

These exams are for the purposes of comparison with others of the same type performed in series or within a reasonable period of time: for example, in the first case, thoracic X-rays of

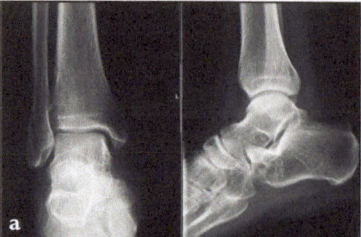

Compound spiral fracture of the peroneal malleolus. The articular connections are maintained.

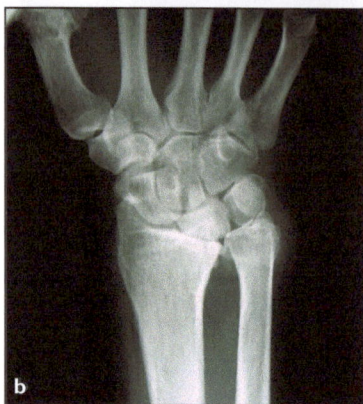

No osseous focal lesions. Arthrosis of the wrist joint with reduction of the articular space between radius and carpus and sclerosis.

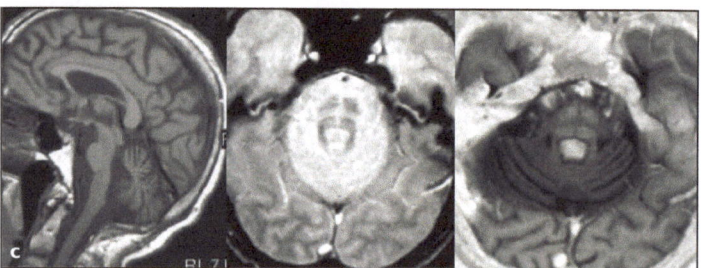

MR examination carried out for suspected extrapyramidal syndrome. [...] One can see atrophy of the pons and of the cerebellum. Transverse signal alterations within the pons. [...]
The picture is suggestive for olivo-ponto-cerebellar atrophy (multisystem atrophy).

Fig. 22 a-c. Examples of first radiological reports on an patient previously unknown to the radiology department or referred for new clinical indications. **a** X-rays of the right ankle at the casualty department for trauma. **b** X-ray of the right wrist due to articular pain. **c** Magnetic resonance of the brain required by a neurologist for suspected extrapyramidal syndrome

a patient in the reanimation department or follow-up of a treated neoplasia (Fig. 23a); in the second case, evaluation of the level of evolution of a pulmonary nodule (Fig. 23b) or of a known osteoarticular pathology (Fig. 20).

In this case, the report must consider the previous exams, signaling either stability of the known situation or its modifications, but neglecting the rest, particularly ex novo interpretations, which are not required. There are two things to be said about this type of report. First, the radiologist must have not just the images, but also – perhaps especially – the report of the previous exam. It must be remembered that the report always expresses the subjective interpretation of the radiologist, this aspect being generally neglected by all (patients, prescribers, and services alike). Second, the reporter must be reasonably certain that the radiological situation being compared is known to

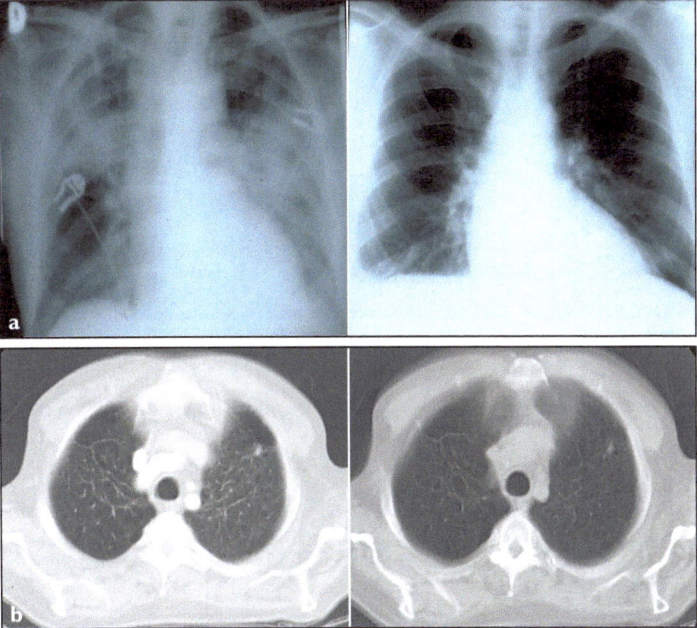

Fig. 23 a, b. Medical reports of control tests, with others carried out within a reasonable timeframe. **a** Control of congestive heart failure in a patient hospitalized in intensive care. **b** Control of a pulmonary nodule after 6 months

the prescriber, who otherwise may not understand the meaning of second the report (if, for example, the prescriber is not the one who prescribed the previous exam). But these aspects are, at least partly, about to be eliminated by PACS, which provides reports online (see chapter "Structured Reports and PACS"). In both cases, the radiologist's sensitivity (see next chapter) or negligence will decide the report's quality and effectiveness.

ADDITIONAL EXAM

These are for the purpose of integrating previous exams performed for the same clinical reason but were not exhaustive; that is, unforeseen incidental reports that are inevitably incomplete. In the first case, this could be a three-phase CT for characterizing a focal lesion to the liver seen on a standard ultrasound scan (Fig. 24a). In the second case, a it could be a CT confirming a pulmonary nodule seen on a thoracic X-ray performed for anesthesiological reasons (Fig. 24b). In this case,

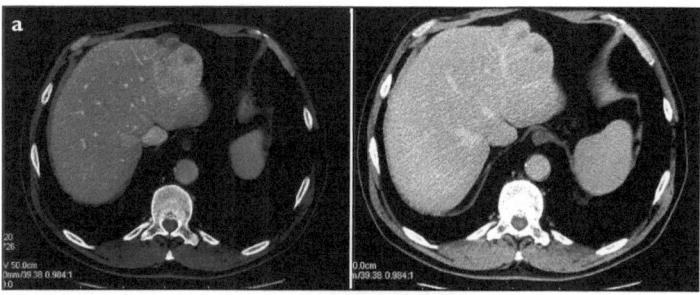

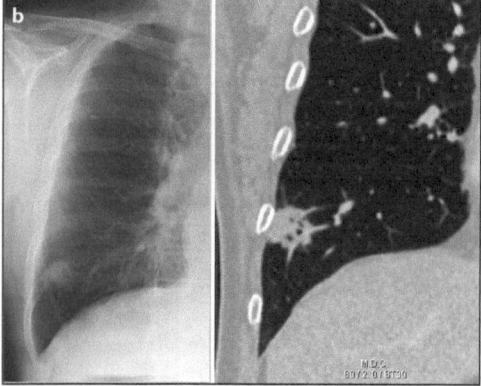

Fig. 24 a, b. In the report, the reasons for these diagnostic in-depth examinations must be explained, pointing out the exhibits that are useful in order to clarify the suspicions not yet solved. **a** Computed tomography integration examinations performed to characterize a hepatic lesion **b** and a pulmonary nodule (bronchioloalveolar carcinoma)

the report must necessarily refer to the previous exam(s) – especially to that/those requiring integration – confirming known elements and, especially, clarifying obscure points, in respect of the sequential nature of the exams.

Of course, this type of report has an even greater need of the previous material and, equally, the specialist's understanding of the clinical and/or radiological issues to be solved (see chapter "From the Typology of the Report to the Sensitivity of the Radiologist"). This is important to the extent that – in order to obtain excellent results – the best thing would be to use the same radiologist as the one who performed the previous exams and is already aware of the case and, possibly, had requested the integration. The alternative – which is not always guaranteed or a foregone conclusion! – is dialogue between colleagues.

PREVENTIVE EXAM

The preventive exam is performed on a healthy person, generally within the sphere of preventive programs (e.g., breast cancer).

In this case, the type of communication is based on the fact that the subjects are not patients, that is, people who do not feel well. They are users, that is, people who feel well. Not only does this affect the report, but – more generally speaking – the type of relationship that is established. It is no longer a relationship of subjection of the weak and suffering patient toward the specialist, but one of equality, as the user is in perfect health at the moment of the exam. This implies that the user is in a physical and psychological position to demand accurate information and respectful treatment, and that the radiologist can wield a very strong power, sufficient to severely disrupt the life of that person by issuing the report.

As regards the first aspect, the difference can already be perceived at the front office. When a user comes to book the exam, is advised to make an appointment in a screening program, collects the report, or is informed of an extension of the exam, that user will not tolerate mediocrity; that is, the slightest mistake or error of communication (Fig. 25).

The second aspect will be discussed later, but one can anticipate the contents of the discussion given that the user/radiologist relationship is one of equality and thus the radiologist

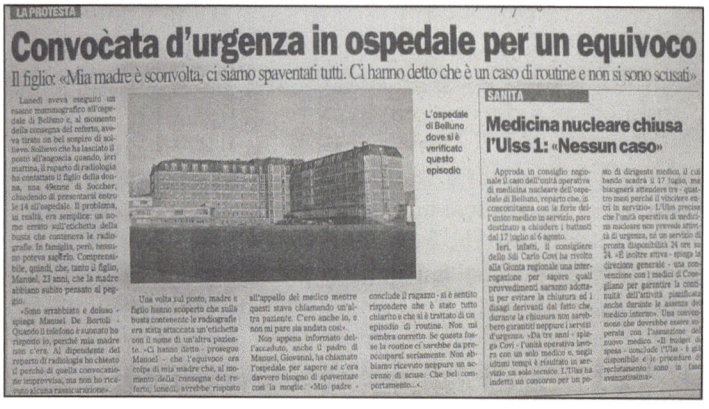

Called urgently to hospital for misunderstanding.
The son: "My mother is shocked, we are scared to death! They told us –
'it is a routine case!' and didn't give us the reasons for being called back".

Fig. 25. Communication errors to the front office are not acceptable. A complaint letter sent to the local newspaper in which the user's son complains about a lack of information as to why his mother was re-called the day after a mammogram, convinced she was about to be given bad news when it was only a question of correcting a data error

has no excuse for being inadequate. In this case, the report will be much more schematic and simple than in other situations: absence of illness with an appointment for the subsequent exam (Fig. 26a); identification of signs of illness with immediate implementation of the relative procedures (Fig. 26b); discovery of situations that need to be analyzed through level-2 exams (Fig. 26c).

SYNTHESIS VERSUS ANALYSIS?

We have often discussed the basic problem concerning the general layout of the report structure: must it be analytical or synthetic?

It is not easy to find a solution that is definitive and valid for every case. By definition, an analytical report is very detailed. It does not just indicate the elements connected with pathologies or lesions but tends to reveal every other signifi-

a

No suspect elements found. Next check up in 2 years.

b

In the upper-lateral quadrant of the right breast there is a speculated nodular formation, interesting for neoproliferative lesion. [...] A histologic examination for the diagnostic confirmation and a surgery evaluation are needed.

c

In the upper-lateral quadrant of the right breast there is a suspicious parenchymatous distortion in an area of 1,5 cm – with point microcalcifications in the context. A diagnostic in-depth examination is needed, with cyto-histologic examination.

Fig. 26 a-c. Mammography reports in which the radiologist's skill determines the patient's clinical history and quality of life

cant detail. The analytical report closely follows the mechanism of decomposition performed on the image by the radiologist's eye. However, due to this excessive redundancy, the analytical report may be dispersive for those who read it and not immediately clear for its recipient. The decisive information, that to which attention should be drawn, may escape readers, and its importance may be underestimated.

Sometimes, therefore, a more synthetic type of communication may be necessary. The conceptual and communicative synthesis is expressed in the capacity of collecting and condensing a great deal of data into a single piece of information. In short, the fundamental meaning of the report is put in the foreground: what is important is said immediately and with fewer words. The advantage of this kind of reporting is evident: it saves time and effort for the reader and the listener, allowing them to immediately understand the contents of the communication. But there are also disadvantages. The first is superficiality. Synthesis is generally less precise and less descriptive. It is forced to neglect certain details that may sometimes be important. Second, it is by no means certain that an element that in the reporter's judgment appears secondary may, on the contrary, be of primary interest to other people. Hence, the danger of underestimation that a bad synthesis can generate.

What can we do then? We believe that analysis and synthesis in a report do not rule each other out. A report that is too analytical can generate the same dangers as a report that is too synthetic. Similarly, to all conceptual and linguistic instruments, analysis and synthesis must be measured by a good radiologist depending on circumstances, type of lesion or pathology, general state of the patient, and according to other elements that the radiologist alone – by virtue of experience and culture – knows how to assess.

to all previous material – images and reports – in order to put the exam into perspective and to understand the case. In these two types of exam, the radiologist's sensitivity involves respect for the work of other professionals and the patience to interpret that work. The radiologist must carefully read and understand the previous report(s) so that the person reading the new report – the doctor in charge – can see that the radiologist has paid respect to the work of other professionals by taking into account the patient's radiological history; it can be seen that the exam is not simply extemporary.

Too often, (even among members of the same team!), paying respect to other professionals' work does not exist. This results in the correct sequence not being respected, interpretations being attributed to a colleague that he or she did not make, or not giving due consideration to interpretations that a colleague did make (Fig. 27). This can be due to superficiality, inattention, or – worse – the desire to appear important, all to the detriment of other people by not respecting the logical sequence of the exams and, therefore, the clinical requirements for which the exam was requested.

In follow-up exams, the radiologist is basically required to make a comparison with the previous exam, with some pre-

a *[...] from L2 to S1, degenerative discopathy with a moderate posterior displacement of the discs, in a type of "bulging anulus"; however, without any evident effect on the dural sac and the lateral canal. In particular, there are no signs of herniated discs.*

b *Compared with the previous test dated...,* we can see an increase in volume of the central hernia L3–L4 and of the left lateral hernia L2-L3 ... *Otherwise, the clinical picture remains unchanged.*

Fig. 27 a, b. Medical reports in which the second report is not in line with what was previously reported by a colleague, either ascribing to him or her interpretations that were not made or not taking into consideration what he or she had written. **a** Report: magnetic resonance (MR) of the lumbar column (first radiologist). **b** Report: MR of the lumbar column (control – second radiologist)

Chapter 7
From the Typology of the Report to the Sensitivity of the Radiologist

---

A fair level of sensitivity in the radiologist is fundamental for report quality. The report – as previously stated – is nothing more than an official opinion, a subjective interpretation, and as such, is influenced by the radiologist's character. As a result, after reading many reports from the same structure, some prescribers can recognize the radiology specialist from his or her style alone, without having to read the name or initials, so strong is the author's character. In turn, the various types of reports require different levels of sensitivity.

INITIAL EXAM
In the initial exam, it is sufficient to follow the conventional report layout and do it as well as possible. This type of report gives more value to the professionalism than to the sensitivity of the radiologist. For this reason, memorized phrases or preprinted reports can compensate for a radiologist's mediocrity, placing him or her within the limits of acceptability, but they can also be detrimental if the radiologist has the skill to produce better reports. It is a little like the political marks required by students during the legendary season of 1968: it does not penalize mediocrity, but neither does it reward skill. In other words, it flattens.

FOLLOW-UP AND ADDITIONAL EXAMS
There are, however, other types of reports that highlight the radiologist's sensitivity and give it a predominant role. In follow-up and additional exams, the radiologist must have access

cautions (as mentioned in the chapter "Principal Report Typologies"). The radiologist must perceive whether the prescriber is the same person who prescribed the previous exam or,
at least, has access to the report. On this basis, the report must
be modulated by selecting the appropriate option. That might
mean drawing up a complete report if it is considered that the
prescriber is not aware of the patient's previous condition (making sure, however, to indicate at the end of the report whether
or not the situation remains unchanged, as the follow-up exam
is always a comparative exam). Or if it is considered that the
prescriber is aware of the patient's previous condition, it might
mean drawing up a concise report that only describes whether
or not the radiological situation remains unaltered.

For additional exams, the radiologist must understand the
clinical and/or radiological context that made that exam necessary, select the most appropriate technique for expressing it,
and define the uncertainty that initiated the exam.

The substantial difference between the two types of exams
lies at the clinical level: in the follow-up exam, comparison
with the previous exam prevails (Fig. 23), whereas the additional exam focuses on evaluating the clinical problem or the
diagnostic uncertainty (Fig. 24). In both cases, the respect of
the radiologist is expressed not only toward the work of other
professionals, but also toward the radiological history of the
patient by maintaining its continuity and logical connection.

PREVENTIVE EXAMS

The dynamics of preventive exams are totally different. The report is simple because the exam is basically a test: in this case,
in fact, certain incidental reports – such as cystic dystrophy in
the prevention of breast cancer or banal isolated pleural plates
in lung cancer – can just be elements of confusion and, as
such, are not appreciated. In these exams, the radiologist's sensitivity depends on oral communication skills, as professionalism is connected not only with the interpretation of the exam
but also, and especially, with the method of transmitting the
result when it is necessary to do so. In fact, no other situation
is as effective in revealing the radiologist's power, which we
have already discussed: that is, the faculty of drastically affecting the life of a person who thinks he or she is healthy.

Communication is certainly more effective when it is free from emotional elements, both from the radiologist and from the user/patient. In the first case, a radiologist with a weak personality may be conditioned by the patient's anxiety and not know how to address it. The radiologist may, for example, decide not to perform an additional mammogram in the event of a possible lesion or not to call the patient to complete the exam, thus letting the correct diagnosis escape. In the second case, it is appropriate from time to time to think about how and with whom to communicate: in fact, communication is not always most effective with the interested party but may be better if performed through a family member. Generally speaking, therefore, in the case of the child, one communicates with the parent; in the case of an elderly person, with the son (making sure the son is not too emotionally involved, otherwise it is best to communicate with an intermediate and acquired relative, such as a brother-in-law, daughter-in-law, etc.); in the case of an adult, directly with that person. Faced with all these options, it is up to the radiologist to decide upon the best one: an incorrect or inadequate choice can have serious consequences (Fig. 25).

Chapter 8

The Psychology of a Good Report: Radiologist and User

As mentioned in the previous chapter, a good-quality report requires an equally good sensitivity on the part of the radiologist. This applies to all types of reports, with the partial exclusion of the initial exam.

In the initial exam, the radiologist expresses professionalism to the utmost: previous documents need not be evaluated nor other reports interpreted. It simply requires understanding the clinical request and basing the report on it. Therefore, at the most, the radiologist must respect the uncertainties and needs of the prescriber, be capable of maintaining independent judgment so as not to be led astray or excessively conditioned, and put the diagnostic process back onto the right track, if necessary (Fig. 28).

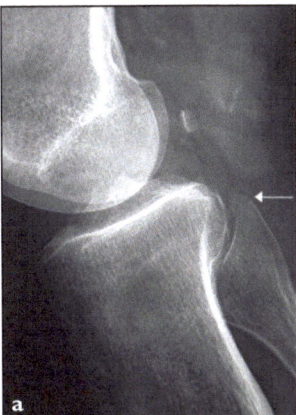

b
[…] in the lateral projection, one can see an image of a fissure of the proximal extremity of the peroneal bone, suggesting a compound fracture.

Fig. 28 a, b. In this case, a wrong clinical analysis is corrected by the radiologist, who must maintain autonomy of judgment to put the diagnostic–therapeutic process back on the right track: the X-ray was requested for gonalgia, without mentioning the trauma previously suffered by the patient. **a** X-ray of the right knee. **b** Report requested for gonalgia

In all the other cases, the report must always respect some-one if it wishes to be correct, of good quality, and clinically valid: professionals – radiologists, prescribers, and other specialists in follow-up and "additional" exams, and users in preventive exams.

Therefore, if we wish to synthesize the relationship between sensitivity and professionalism for a good report – on the basis of the above-mentioned types of report – we could say that more professionalism than sensitivity is required in the initial exam, whereas they are equivalent in the others, with both playing a very important role (Table 2).

It should be pointed out, however, that – as with all other medical acts – the report must give priority to the interest of the patient and/or user, who among other things – in medical-legal terms – is the final recipient and holder. This means that there can be no ambiguities in the preventive exam, as there is a direct relationship between the radiologist and the user; in other words, there are no intermediaries, such as the prescriber. However, in follow-up and additional exams, the interests of the patient and of the radiologist may conflict. An example would be a misunderstood fracture or a blatantly missed radiological diagnosis (Fig. 29) to the extent that the reporter cannot always reconcile the conflict but must make a choice, obviously in favor of the patient.

Though emphasizing that the work of other professionals must always be respected, basic or specific incompetence cannot be covered up if this means a missing or incomplete diagnosis. As is logical, it is up to the radiologist's sensitivity to use terms or expressions that soften the impact, such as: "In today's examination, performed as an integration of the previous one…"; or "Following today's exam based on detailed radiographs…" (Fig. 30).

On the contrary, it may also be true that due to an incorrect interpretation in favor of the patient's health or for the possi-

Table 2. Incidence of Sensitivity and Professionality in the X-ray Report

	First test	Control	Integration	Prevention
Sensitivity	++	+++	+++	+++
Professionality	++++	+++	+++	+++

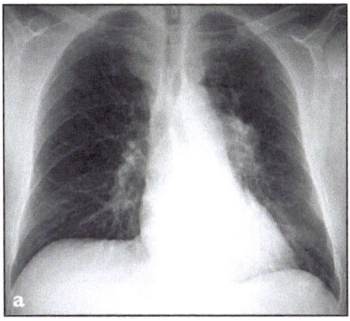

b
Pulmonary infiltrations are not shown.
The vascular pattern is marked, mainly on the left hilum.

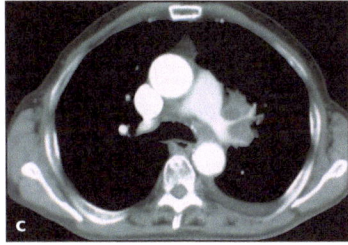

d
[...] heteroplastic lesion of the pulmonary hilum on the left, which infiltrates the adjacent bronchial-vascular structures [...]

Fig. 29 a-d. Control test in which pulmonary computed tomography (CT) is carried out following an X-ray of the thorax in which the radiologist blatantly misses the diagnosis. In this case, the medical report of the CT must necessarily disprove the previous report. **a** X-ray of the thorax. **b** Report: thorax X-ray 25/05/07. **c** CT of the lungs. **d** Report: CT of the thorax 20/06/07

bility of appearing important, the reporter may equally as blatantly prove the colleague wrong (Fig. 31) or add elements to the report that are totally insignificant from the diagnostic point of view purely for the purpose of distinguishing himself or herself (Fig. 32). All this emphasizes how protection of the patient and of the professional team is not an easy objective to attain.

Another distinctive quality of a radiologist is a good personality: a firm belief in himself or herself. Everyone often has uncertainties and doubts about a case that is not conclusive and, on the basis of the principle that four eyes are better than two, wishes to be comforted by the opinion of a trusted colleague. In this case, we are psychologically prepared to consider his or her opinion as correct and to take it into account in our report.

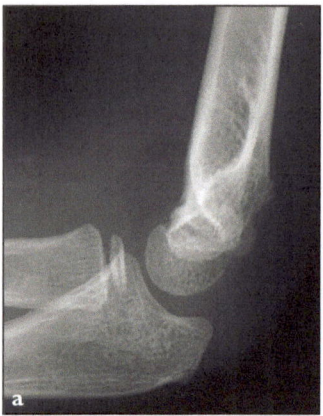

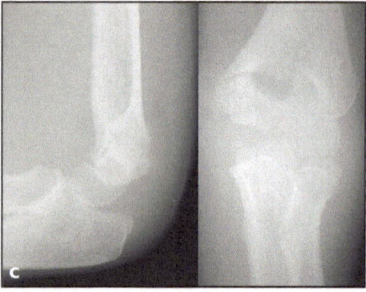

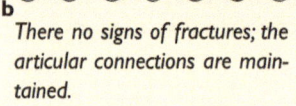

There no signs of fractures; the articular connections are maintained.

This is a control test that was carried out because the symptoms have not disappeared (pain and reduced function): from today's examination, having carried out further X-rays in detail, a fissure of compound over-condyloid fracture can be identified.

Fig. 30 a-d. A case of diagnostic error, which is corrected in the following control through a choice of wording that does not put the previous colleague in a difficult position. **a** First X-ray of the right elbow. **b** Report: first examination 20/05/07. **c** Second X-ray of the right elbow. **d** Report: second examination 20/06/07

Similarly, in follow-up and additional exams, just as the radiologist can more or less correctly and appropriately disprove the report of the preceding radiologist, he or she can equally submit to the predecessor's influence – considering that professional to be expert, reliable, and charismatic – to the point of persisting with any errors that predecessor made (Fig. 33). This is further confirmation of the fact that whereas the report is the work of a single person, it is also the outcome of multiple and often interdisciplinary evaluations. Not only do all these psychological and behavioral aspects – superficiality, inattention, incorrect behavior between colleagues, psychological subjection – harm the image of these doctors and the services in which they function, they can also expose them to medical-legal risks (Fig. 34).

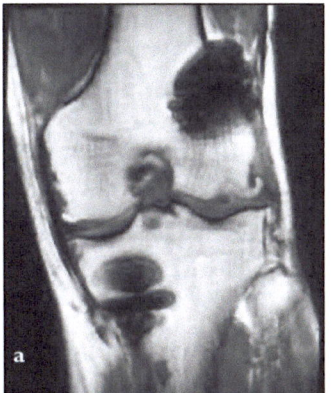

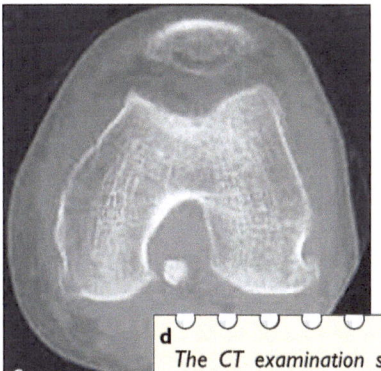

b
End results of the reconstruction of the frontal cruciate ligament. There is an alteration in the signal from the femoral-tibial cartilage and from the subchondral bone, compatible with osteochondritis...

d
The CT examination shows a loose bone fragment located posteriorly into the intercondyloid fossa. [...]
This bone fragment was already present at the time of the previous MR examination, as one can see on DP axial and sagittal images ...

Fig. 31 a-d. Thi[...] occasional inability to walk and has already u[...] ruction of the frontal cruciate ligament. A [...] ee is then carried out, and the report descri[...] pecially affecting the articular cartilages, bu[...] h is, instead, recognized in the subsequent c[...] ation. The problem is that in medical report[...] bone fragment was already present at the time of the MR and thus points out the mistake made by a colleague. Medical reports of this sort are contrary to the spirit of teamwork because, even if the main objective remains accurate diagnosis and patient interest, there are many ways of getting there. Probably, there is no intention of damaging a colleague, but only aspiration to "show off". Regardless, this is a dangerous approach that could undermine the credibility of a colleague and encourage, instead, a proliferation of court cases. Perhaps in such cases it would be better to opt for a collegial revision of the reports, dealing with the crisis as a group, to contain or at least limit medical reports of this sort – as it would be too much to hope to abolish them. **a** MR of the left knee. **b** Report: first examination. **c** CT of the left knee. **d** Report: second (control) examination

a

On the right, we can observe the end results of a nodulectomy in the superolateral quadrant, without current evident elements of suspicion. On the left, the mammography remains unchanged, without any evident lesion. The echographic control does not show, at present, on either side any active focal lesion.

b

The mammography shows, in the superoexternal area of the right breast, a parenchymal distortion – partly already present at the time of the previous examination – of about 2 cm in diameter, which reaches the skin, which has been thickened by the treatment. [...]

Given the history of the patient, a further investigation through a needle biopsy is recommended.

c

[...] Fragments of fibroadipose and striated muscular tissue, without significant morphological changes.

Fig. 32 a-c. Misinterpretation, either of caring for the patient or of an opportunity to look better than one's colleague. The doctor writing the control report adds elements of uncertainty, doubting the first diagnostic interpretation, and the patient subsequently undergoes a supplementary invasive test, which is superfluous. **a** Medical report from the first doctor: clinical-instrumental examination of the breast. **b** Medical report (control) from the second doctor: clinical–instrumental exam of the breast. **c** Medical report in reference to needle biopsy (third test): histopathological report

Another aspect that should not be undervalued is pathos; that is, the emotion of the radiologist when drawing up the report, which must be perceived by the prescriber. In fact, giving a structure and a precise method to the report serves to allow the prescriber to have faith in the radiologist's seriousness; equally, giving the report a certain warmth gives an impression of the reporter's commitment and participation in writing it. This is very useful in complex cases where the prescriber may come across difficulties of interpretation (Fig. 35). In a report drawn up in a cold and aseptic manner (Fig. 36) in which the clinical motivation is only hinted at and the rest is made up of memorized phrases, one can only communicate the sensation of an assembly made without any personality.

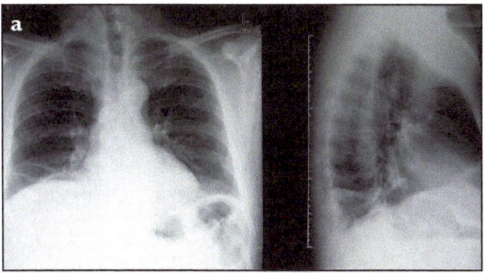

b

Urgent request made by the casualty department because of pain in the lower right hemithorax, with a temperature: infiltration on the right lung? Right hemidiaphragm slightly elevated, with some stria likely to be fibrotic at the bottom right. The costophrenic angles and not very deep. There is no pleural effusion. *Hila and heart are within the limits.*

c

... On the right, at the height of the posterior segment of the right inferior lobe, one can see an area of ground-glass opacity associated with fibrotic stria departing from the pleura and a pleural effusion of moderate consistency. ...

d

Compared with the previous test dtd. 03/06/09, we can observe that the right pulmonary basis appears clearer; there are still traces of pleural effusion with posterior costophrenic angle obliteration. There is nothing noteworthy on the left side; the mediastinum is within its normal limits.

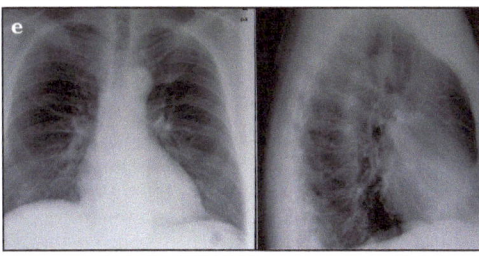

Fig. 33 a-e. A medical report drawn up by a colleague believed to be more competent could influence a younger doctor to the point of continuing an error. In the first report, on the radiological examination of the chest, a highly respected radiologist on the team mistakes the disventilatory bands at the base of the right pulmonary field with fibrotic results. In the subsequent computed tomography (CT) examination, a young radiologist, obviously very impressionable, gives the same interpretation. Frontal radiograph of the latest check examination and relative report show the disappearance of what was found and described the earlier reports. **a** Frontal radiography of the chest. **b** Medical report from the first radiologist, 03/09/06. **c** Medical report from the second, and younger, radiologist: CT of the thorax 05/09/06. **d** Frontal radiograph of the latest check examination. **e** Medical report from the third examination: X-ray of the thorax 21/09/06

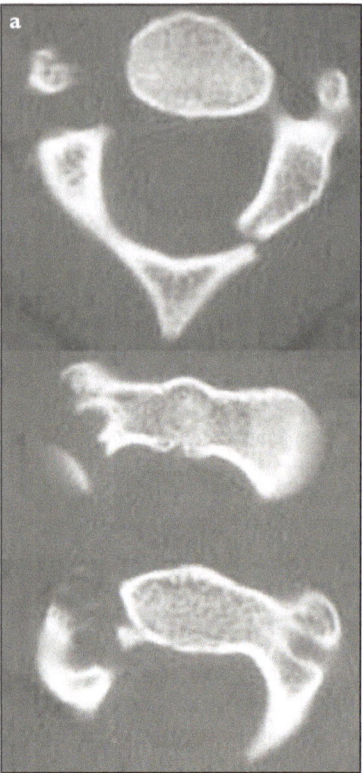

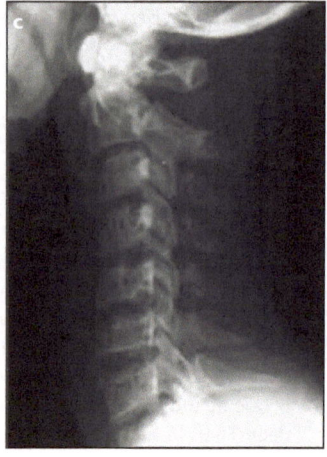

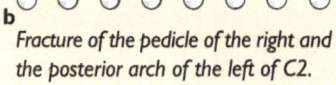

b
Fracture of the pedicle of the right and the posterior arch of the left of C2.

d
There are no previous examinations available to make a comparison.
Mild anterolisthesis of C2 on C3. The pedicle of C2 seems to be interrupted and partially overlapping. No further traumatic alterations are evident.
The picture is compatible with an unstable fracture of the posterior arch of C2 (Hangman) with a slight anterior sliding of C2 on C3.

Fig. 34 a-d. Here there is a double error: one deriving from insufficient professional expertise and one determined by an insufficient psychological profile. The first doctor issues a medical report for a computed tomography (CT), which is extremely brief and insufficient, being referred to as a traumatic vertebral lesion, however, on evaluation by a neurosurgeon. The second doctor describes an extremely detailed clinical picture following radiological control of the cervical column. However, this second report highlighted further findings, which had not been identified during the previous CT, generating alarm for the patient, who is later "reassured" by the neurosurgeon. The second doctor did not follow test sequence and/or integration. This failing communicates confusion and uncertainty and is also dangerous from the point of view of legal liability. **a** CT of the cervical spine. **b** Brief report cervical spine CT 15/09/05: issued by the first radiologist. **c** X-ray of the cervical column. **d** Report of control X-ray (18/10/05): issued by the second radiologist

a

Preoperative prostatectomy checkup.
... Two suspicious inhomogeneously hypodense areas can be observed on the liver, whose dimensions are respectively 5 and 2 cm. ...

b

Examination required to complete the preceding CT examination of ...
The presence of two nodular hepatic formations is confirmed. The major one, level with the right lobe and with a diameter of about 5 cm and in-homogeneous signal, is hypointense in the T1 basal sequences with sub-tle hypointense rim, inhomogeneously hyperintense in T2, with signal enhancement in the peripheral area after gadolinium, and low intrale-sional enhancement even in the late sequences. The second lesion, level with the left lobe and with a diameter of 2 cm, shows a clear and ho-mogeneous signal enhancement in arterial stage, small hyperintensity in balance phase, and isointensity in end phase.
Signal characteristics and the contrastographic behavior of the lesions are doubtful and not typical for benign formation or with secondary le-sion pathologies. On the contrary, they are suspicious for primitive he-patic lesions (HCC).

Fig. 35 a, b. The report must be formulated in a technically correct manner, though without being too synthetic or employing memorized phrases, especially in the most complex cases. **a** Medical report: computed tomography of the abdomen. **b** Medical report: hepatic magnetic resonance (same patient)

Oncological checkup.
The CT pattern is unchanged in comparison with the previous ones.

Fig. 36. Too synthetic and aseptic a report, which shows insufficient care by the reporter and produces uncertainty in the prescriber

The harder the radiologist works at providing a clinical de-scription to the diagnostic exam – as described in the chapter "Considerations on the Usefulness of the Clinical Description" – the more appropriate it is to show appreciation for the re-port. In short, just as memorized phrases must not stifle the imagination, structure must not reduce the pathos.

After exploring the most appropriate psychology required by the radiologist to make a good report, it is also beneficial to investigate the psychology of the subject of the communication; that is, the user. The psychology of the person who requests a radiological exam is dominated by what one could define as a feeling of informed expectation. Very often, in the widespread culture of prevention, a person who enters a hospital has been sent there by the family doctor or a specialist after requesting additional investigation with respect to symptoms that could signify a pathological state. This could be seen not as passive but as active behavior, in many cases due to the increased capacity of the general public to identify a possible problem requiring a response. In some cases, this also goes hand in hand with a precise memory of the results of previous findings and a discreet availability of anamneses with respect to present and past conditions, which increase the user's expectation of equally efficient service from the doctor.

However, the feeling that dominates the user's behavior is that of expectation for communication that should settle a problematic situation and open up new prospects for the future. The expectation can, in fact, either end up in relief, thanks to a favorable report, or turn into anguish, in the case of an unfavorable response. Between the two possible outcomes lies the communication of the radiologist who, knowing the outcome in advance, must accept the burden of determining, above all, the second. In this difficult situation, the doctor's communication and the user's understanding may be imprecise and vague. We must ask ourselves: is this kind of language in the interest of the person who asked for the service? Does it correspond to the active and often competent method with which the person requested the exam and collected the report? Above all, if we assume that the structure of the doctor-patient/user relationship is less hierarchic and more equal, will we, the patient/user or radiologist, accept that our peer, in this case the doctor, treats us like an "inferior", talking to us vaguely or hiding something from us? We would say no: and then, for an elementary rule of uniformity, we must wish for ourselves and for others that every communication concerning people's physical integrity is based on outstanding clarity and competence.

Chapter 9
Radiological Semiotics in the Report

A coarse, macroscopic report can be understood by anyone: this bears out the curiosity and presumed competence with which many clinicians examine the so-called plates against the light or indicate the report with their fingers on the diaphanoscope or the monitor (Fig. 37). It is a custom that has always existed and will always exist, because diagnostic images attract people, especially nowadays when we have pan-explorative methods and submicroscopic details; so much so, in fact, that the radiologist has always been labeled more as the producer – the photographer – than as the reporter.

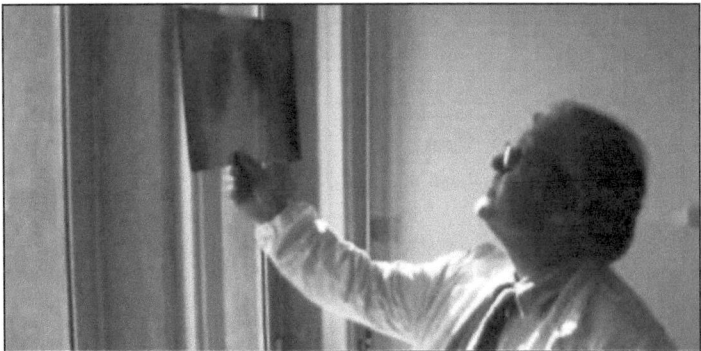

Fig. 37. Many clinicians who claim to have better specific competence than the radiologist (for example, odontologists, orthopedists, pneumologists) believe that they are able to interpret the examination backlit in the window, without even having read the report. It is up to the radiologist's professionalism – the good report! – to win their trust

Only with a well-written report that affects the treatment or subsequent development to the exact diagnosis does the radiologist maintain a clinical role (Fig. 38). Conversely, with insufficient (Fig. 39) or remiss reports (Fig. 40), the radiologist leaves the reading and practical interpretation to others, namely, the prescribing physician.

How does the radiologist express his or her specific professionalism? Only by knowing how to use his or her semiotics, comprising direct and indirect signs. Therefore, when faced with a gross plurisegmentary pneumonia parenchymal thickening in an adult/elderly person – perhaps a smoker or an ex-smoker – the radiologist must consider the possibility that it is the epiphenomenon of a bronchial neoplastic obstruction and therefore evaluate – and express it in the report –

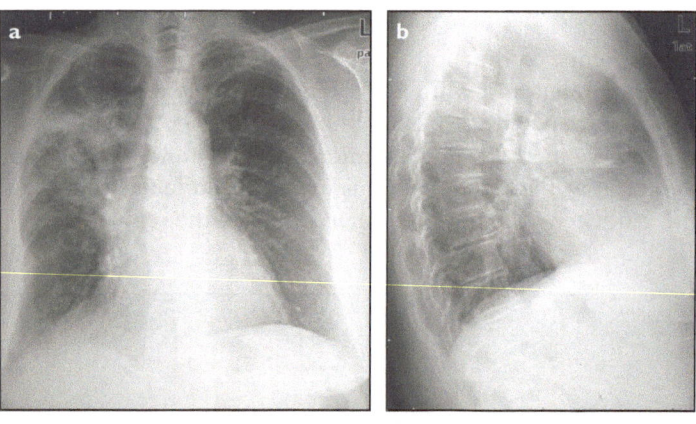

c *Request made because of temperature, cough, and pain in the upper right abdomen.*
Extensive consolidation in right upper lobe with mild upward bulge of displaced minor fissure. Right hilum appears enlarged and increased in density. [...]
Conclusion: pneumonia with partial lobar atelectasis, which needs further investigation.

Fig. 38 a-c. Good report that considers both direct and indirect pathological signs, with a positive effect on the definition of the clinical situation. **a** Chest X-ray: frontal view. **b** Chest X-ray: lateral view. **c** Medical report

whether or not it is accompanied by loss of volume. Doing so necessitates considering all the indirect signs that should be known to the radiologist but not necessarily to other clinicians (retraction of the mediastinum; movement of the clefts, of the

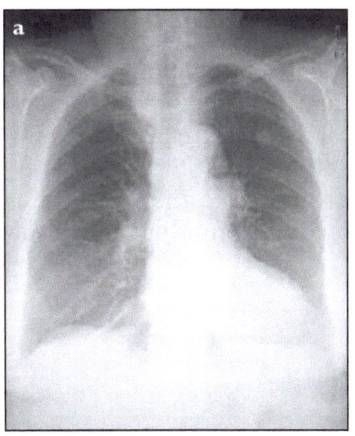

b

... There is a dense rounded, opacity projecting into the posterior arch of the VI rib on the left (bone callous following a trauma?) ...

d

The CT examination, carried out following a previous X-ray of the thorax dtd..., shows a nodule of the left upper lobe...

Fig. 39 a-d. An insufficient medical report in which the opacity of the left hemithorax is not correctly interpreted with a more detailed scan or through a radioscopic control, as shown in the subsequent computed tomography (CT). **a** X-ray of the thorax. **b** First and insufficient report: X-ray of the thorax. **c** CT of the thorax. **d** Second report: thorax CT

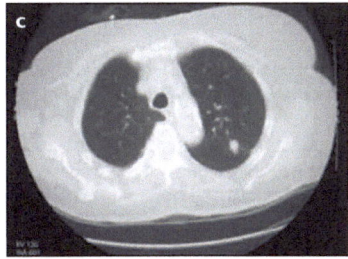

Control of hip arthroprosthesis: the images sent to the referring specialist for viewing.

Fig. 40. Report: X-ray of the right hip. A medical report in which the radiologist relinquishes his or her role and delegates interpretation to the orthopedic specialist

hilus, of the hemidiaphragm; rarefaction of the vascular pattern in the residue lung, etc.). This allows the radiologist to issue the diagnostic suspicion and recommend the subsequent exam, that is, the bronchoscopy (Fig. 41). Or, again in the sphere of the chest, the radiologist must be able to distinguish the exact seat of an epiphrenic opacity (parenchymal or extraparenchymal, of the omental or Bochdalek hernia type) (Fig. 42); or in the case of a patient sent due to prevailingly nocturnal coughing, to understand the cause and be able to describe all signs of congestion of the small region due to initial insufficiency in the left side of the heart (Fig. 43). It is evident that in this case, a report limited to the presence or absence of active pneumopulmonary lesions is not only insuf-

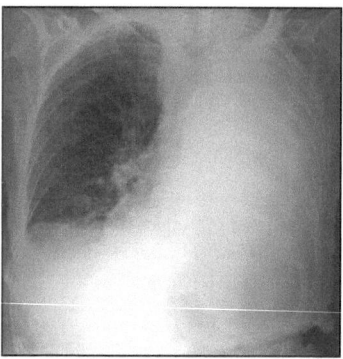

Fig. 41. The thorax radiological semiotic guides the diagnostic process, as in this case where the left hemithorax is completely opaque. There is no view of the principal homolateral bronchus, and there is homolateral retraction of the mediastinum, which suggest further investigation through a bronchoscopy should be carried out

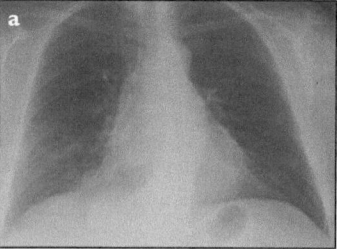 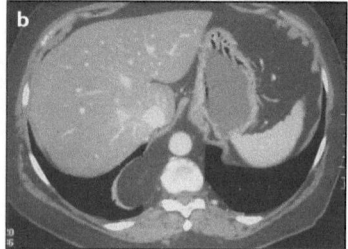

Fig. 42 a, b. Diagnostic sign that only the radiologist is able to interpret. The radiological examination of the chest shows a bosselation of the posterior right hemidiaphragm: lesion place and morphology suggest an initial hypothesis of hernia formation, which is then confirmed by the subsequent computed tomography (CT). **a** Chest X-ray, frontal projection. **b** Bochdalek hernia on CT

ficient but also demonstrates the inadequate clinical role of the radiologist.

There are many examples for any organ or sector, all connected with one aspect: the need for the radiologist to understand the clinical problem lying behind the requested diagnostic exam and consequently to choose the best method of performing the exam, describing the situation, and reaching the conclusion. These are all aspects we have already discussed and will be discussed again at a later stage.

It is evident that underevaluation of or failure to understand the request will condition the rest of the process and condemn the radiologist to remain just a photographer for clinicians. Taking the concepts to extremes, we could say that patient semiotics mainly comprises direct signs (lesions, mass subforms, nodules, etc.) and user semiotics comprises indirect signs (convergence, distortion, etc.). In an evolving clinical case, the existence of a pathological situation can be supposed, although this must be confirmed, quantified, and typified. In the preclinical phase, it is more frequent to find situations that

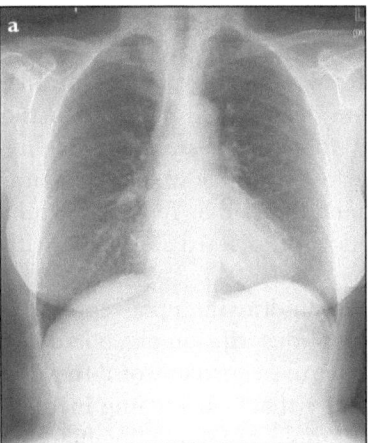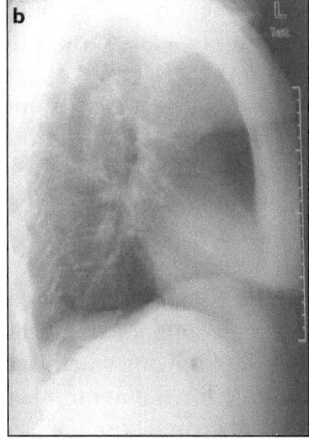

Fig. 43 a, b. In the radiological examination of the thorax, we should not only exclude the presence of pleural–parenchymal lesions but also identify any possible alteration concerning the heart and the pulmonary circle. In this patient, referred because of a "persisting cough, especially at night", signs are visible of overloading of the pulmonary circle due to initial congestive heart failure. **a** Thorax X-ray, frontal projection. **b** Thorax X-ray, lateral projection

are less visible or at the limits of visibility, to the extent that – in prevention programs, in particular (neoplasia of the breast, lung, colon, etc.) – it is necessary to utilize computer supports (CAD). This approach also – different patient and user semiotics – bears out the fact that the patient report must be drawn up in a different way from the user report. The first case is based more on the methodology followed and on the description of the direct signs. The second case is based more on the search for indirect signs.

Returning to the initial image of the clinician with the plate in his hand: we understand how this can happen in the case of a patient who needs clinical management and whose radiological situations are macroscopic and therefore easy for all to see. But this is not so in the case of the user, who has a direct relationship with the radiologist. In the ultimate analysis, the radiologist demonstrates professionalism in the case of the patient when exactly describing and interpreting all the direct and indirect signs, regardless of the opinion of other specialists. In the case of the user, the radiologist's professionalism is demonstrated when identifying those indirect signs that only the specialist can see.

Seeing, on the one hand, the classification of the subjects of radiological exams into users and patients and, on the other, the existence of new totipotent and pan-explorative technology, it is also a question of establishing whether the old semiotics and terminology that describe are suitable for modern-day diagnostic scenarios. In other words, do semiotics and technology still go hand in hand as regards current health needs, or has the second leapt forward compared with the first?

Is it a fact that nowadays, when drawing up a report, the classical signs of the radiological description are borrowed without knowing whether they are used correctly or if they are suitable for the anatomical reality that is becoming increasingly deep and complex? For example, are the fading margins or the structural inhomogeneity of a focal parenchymal lesion described in a CT exam still meaningful?

We should now repeat the observation made by a clinician, Italian broncho-pneumologist Stefano Nardini, at the dawn of CT: "The abandoning of the scopic exam in favor of CT in case

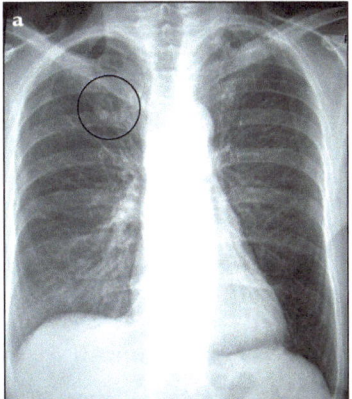

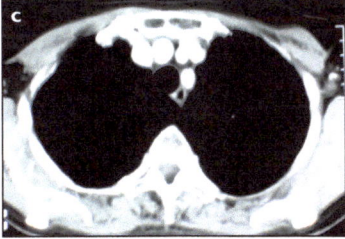
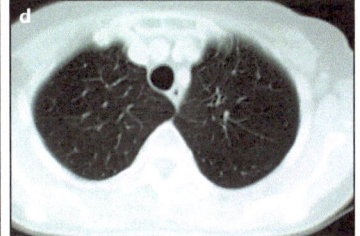

In the right upper lobe, a small opacity can be seen, with a diameter of less than 1 cm and seemingly spiky borders, which needs to be further investigated with a CT of the thorax. ...

Fig. 44 a-d. In this case, abandoning the radiological test in favor of computed tomography (CT) determines the execution of the needless CT, where, for instance the pulmonary nodule being considered is simply the image of the chondrocostal articulation. **a** Thorax X-ray. **b** Report: Interpretation of thorax X-ray. **c, d** CT of the thorax: hypertrophic chondrocostal articulation

of the slightest doubt of traditional radiology (the pulmonary nodule is a classic example) (Fig. 44) can immediately solve the request and solve it well, but it equally deprives the radiologist of his semiotics, what he grew with and what is still taught, at least in Italy – unless it is decided to build a brand new one".

Chapter 10
Considerations on the Usefulness of the Clinical Description

The first element needed to produce a good report is the clinical request, which can be put in the form of diagnostic uncertainty or simple clinical–anamnestic information. The formula that is most appreciated by the radiologist remains to be established, whether the first, which can be insidious and deceptive – as will be described shortly – or the second, which assumes a good clinical basis, especially in the specialist (neurology, pediatrics, geriatrics, etc.) or at least sectorial (hepatology, pneumology, nervous system, etc.) sphere.

However that may be, the need for a well-formulated request has been a controversial subject with the prescriber, but perhaps it is being solved today because the enormous potential of the available methods contrasts with the inadequate behavior of the prescriber. One of the reasons – the most important and unrecognized – requests for diagnostic exams were not accompanied by adequate clinical description was the jealousy of the prescriber, who feared having to abandon his or her prerogatives and who essentially saw the instrumental exam simply as support in the diagnostic strategy implemented by himself or herself. With limited radiological methods, such as those of the past, all this was possible; with current methods, it is not, because they can reveal the inadequacies or errors of the clinicians that preceded them and caused the exam to be requested (Fig. 28). Therefore, it is also a good idea for the prescriber to formulate a good diagnostic request. This will be appreciated not only for his or her sensitivity toward the reporter, but also for his or her good knowledge of modern imaging.

So, why does the radiologist need clinical information? For various reasons:

1. Choosing the most suitable execution technique and study protocol (e.g., a hepatic lesion or a pulmonary nodule to typify, the first using a specific contrast medium and/or three-phase technique; the second using lung-analysis software).

2. Correctly interpreting the reports (for example, finding calcific pulmonary nodules can have a different diagnostic and prognostic significance in a patient suffering from osteosarcoma than in one with tuberculosis).

3. Focusing on essential aspects for a particular pathology (for example, searching for and finding lymphadenomegalies in a CT exam can be essential in a patient who is certainly oenological rather than in one with an exclusively phlogistic pathology).

4. Recommending continuance of the diagnostic path with other exams if the one carried out is not exhaustive (for example, a history of recurrent pneumothorax in a young person may require high-resolution CT scanning for subpleura bubbles if the standard exam is not indicative).

5. Optimizing the cost–benefit ratio of exams, also according to the radiologist's requirements, expressed below.

Therefore, the radiologist should understand from the clinical request the reasons for the exam in order to choose the best way of performing it, provided he or she agrees that this is the most suitable exam. It should not be forgotten that the prescriber simply proposes an exam and the radiologist is exclusively responsible for choosing what type and performing it, with the relative acceptance of clinical and medical–legal responsibility.

Drawing up the report is strictly related to the clinical request, which could affect the report with its strong and its weak points. In the first instance, a good request can be determining for correct radiological diagnosis (Fig. 45); in the second, a too circumstantiated request or the outcome of an incorrect or incomplete objective situation could, in turn, be misleading (Fig. 46). In other words, the clinical description should not limit the radiologist's critical capacities; neither should it overtly condition his or her judgment. The request must be intelligent and open, so as to help the radiologist pres-

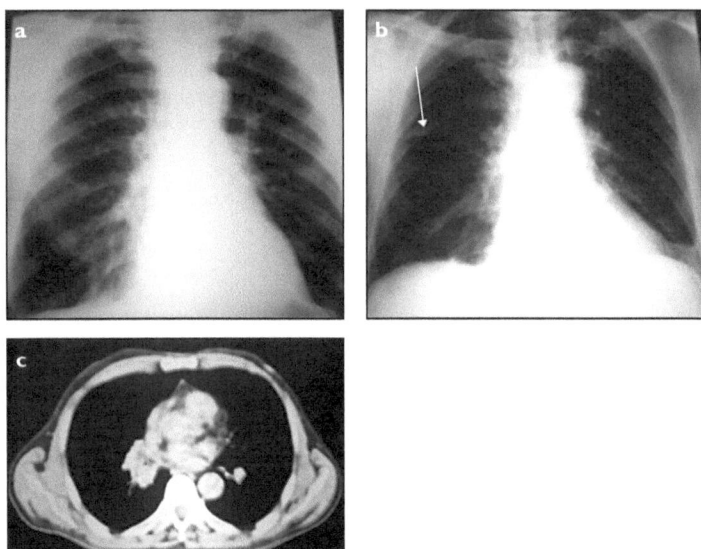

Fig. 45 a-c. A clear clinical suspicion leads the radiologist to choose the best technique to resolve it. Radiography of the thorax is requested for the clinical suspicion of air entrapment at the base of the right lung, producing hyperphonesis on percussion during expiration in auscultation. Therefore, to the standard test of the two projections taken during inspiration, a frontal-projection radiography during expiration is added. Without precise clinical suspicion that suggests radiography should also be taken during expiration, the radiological examination would have resulted as negative, and the diagnosis would only have been made with a bronchoscopy. **a** Frontal-projection radiography taken during inspiration shows a normal clinical picture. **b** Radiography taken during expiration shows the lack of collapse of the lower area in the right pulmonary field (*arrow*). **c** Computed tomography (CT) shows a solid new formation obstructing the bronchus intermedius and causing air entrapment

ent a clinical hierarchy to the report, as will be explained in the chapter "The Rationale of Reporting Methodology."

Some people paradoxically consider that if the radiologist has to choose from two extreme options – a request that is too circumstantiated or one that is practically absent – the latter it is preferable, if only because the radiologist is not excessively conditioned and can more freely describe and interpret everything he or she sees. Regardless, the insufficiency of the clinical request does not excuse the radiologist for making diagnostic errors. Neither does it justify incomplete or inexact reports, because – as we have often stated – the radiologist has

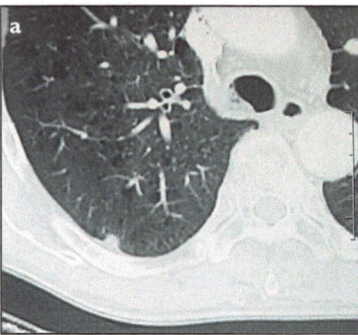

Fig. 46 a-c. A clinical question too clearly oriented toward a diagnostic hypothesis could be misleading for correct interpretation of a radiological examination, as occurred in this case of computed tomography (CT) of the thorax for hemophtoe. **a** CT of the thorax. **b** Report: CT of the thorax. **c** Report: CT of the thorax (control)

b

There are signs of central-lobular emphysema of the upper lobules with a nodule of almost 1 cm adhering to the marginal posterior at the level of the apical segment of the lower lobe. [...]

An irregular thickening of the right posterior-lateral wall of the trachea, in proximity to the bifurcation, substantially at the same level where the nodule is described.

As for the rest, the tomodensitometric picture is within normal limits, as there are no signs of hylomediastinal lymphadenomegalias or pleural effusions.

A bronchoscopy is recommend, together with a clinical-anamnestic evaluation of the above-mentioned nodule.

c

Compared with the previous test dtd..., the nodule adhering to the marginal posterior at the level of the apical segment of the lower lobe is unchanged (this lesion is unchanged also compared with further tests carried out some years ago at a different clinic and brought to us for inspection). The irregularity of the wall that had been noted then in the right posterior-lateral sector in proximity to the bifurcation has now disappeared, being now the regular lumen width.

As for the rest, the tomodensitometric picture is unchanged.

From a radiological point of view, no further examinations are necessary.

full independence and decision-making responsibility in patient management at the same level as other clinicians. This means that as well as choosing the most appropriate type of exam, the radiologist can also refuse to perform it if he or she considers it superfluous and therefore simply harmful and invasive for the patient.

Chapter 11
Common Sense in Clinical and Preclinical Diagnosis

Nowadays, along with totipotent and pan-explorative exams (CT, MR, PET), the traditional exams perform better than in the past due to the improved definition offered by digital technology and the possibility of postprocessing on the monitor. That is, they allow everything that is requested to be seen, and more besides. Therefore, they can equally accurately confirm the clinical suspicion by describing it in essential reports, and they can anticipate a clinical diagnosis itself by describing incidental findings in exams requested for other reasons.

A classic example is ischemic cardiopathy. The coronary calcifications found in a standard thoracic exam can both confirm the clinical situation of insufficiency of the left side of the heart and allow the same diagnosis to be made in the preclinical phase in an at-risk subject (Fig. 47). In the first case, confirmation of the clinical suspicion, the calcification report is essential because it is an integral part of the diagnosis. In the second case, diagnostic anticipation, the reported finding is incidental because the exam was not directly requested. In both cases, however, the report must be expressed with clinical and diagnostic common sense. For example, coronary calcification in a hypertensive 50-year-old smoker is one thing; coronary calcification in a healthy 80-year-old person is another (see the chapter "Normality Reports, Depending on the Subject's Age).

Simplifying to an extreme, the straight-line image, corresponding to the cutoff at the preclinical/clinical phase, may

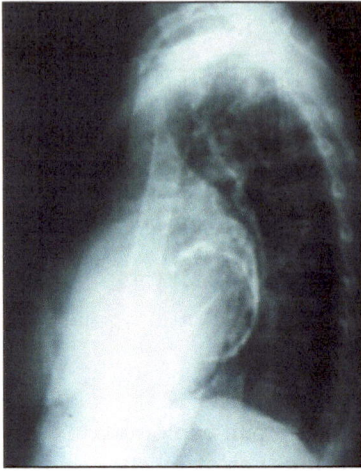

Fig. 47. In the standard radiological test of the thorax, the coronary calcifications detected are an accessory result. However, in the elder patient with signs of heart failure, they represent an integral part of the clinical-radiological picture. In the young patient suffering from asymptomatic hypertension, they represent an incidental finding and could anticipate the clinical diagnosis of ischemic cardiopathy

Table 3. Clinical Utility Simplification of Information

Preclinical diagnosis		**Clinical diagnosis**	
Redundant			Excessive
	EBM	EBM	

be useful (Table 3): all that is outside this in one sense or the other is redundant or useless, as its extension is defined on the basis of evidence-based medicine (EBM).

Chapter 12
The Rationale of Reporting Methodology

This chapter explains the reasons behind the methodology suggested for drawing up the report. Figure 48 shows an example of a typical report for every typology identified, excluding – obviously – preventive exams.

a
The test is carried out for a persistent cough.
No focal parenchymal lesions are evident. The bases are free. The image of the heart is well positioned and within its normal dimensions.

b
Compared with the previous test dtd…, we can observe the onset of a nodular lesion at the right pulmonary basis, of about 1.5 cm. in diameter, with slightly irregular borders. The remaining results are unchanged: in particular, there are no further foci of pulmonary lesions.
The clinical picture requires a further investigation, to be carried out through computed tomography for a clearer definition of the findings.

c
This test was carried out as an integration of the previous radiographic test performed on ….
The nodular lesion noted at the right pulmonary basis of a diameter of about 1.5 cm., showing irregular borders and small internal cavities… The picture suggests a bronchioloalveolar carcinoma.

Fig. 48 a-c. Typical examples from all report typologies, except from a preventive exam. **a** Medical report: X-ray of the thorax, initial exam. **b** Medical report: X-ray of the thorax, control exam. **c** Medical report: computed tomography of the thorax: integrative exam

INITIAL EXAM

Clinical Description
For more information, see the chapter "Considerations on the Usefulness of the Clinical Description". The reasons for inserting the clinical description in the report are summarized in Table 4.

Execution Technique
Execution technique should be mentioned in exams with more than one technical option in order to show that the best decision has been made to solve that clinical request. This is the main principle of clinical radiology [for example, the spectral presaturation with inversion recovery (SPIR) sequence in an MR for a knee distortion or a CT analysis for typifying a pulmonary nodule]. There is no point in doing this when a standardized and known technique and method is used (e.g., convex probe for abdominal ultrasounds or the two orthogonal protections for thoracic X-rays).

Report Description
The report description should be hierarchized on the basis of its clinical impact (for example, in a colon CT, first the description of the tumour and then of the diverticula) and/or the diagnostic suspicion that caused that exam to be requested (for example, always in a colon CT for a suspected neoplasia, first the answer to the clinical request – presence or absence of the lesion – and then the rest). In other words, there must be a hierarchy based on what the prescriber requests and/or what

Table 4. Importance of Clinical Indication in the X-ray Report

– Allows the choice of the right method to solve the clinical problem

– Orients the interpretation of the findings

– Confers logical cohesion to the different parts of the report, thus influencing the conclusions

– Involves the Doctor in charge in the diagnostic event

– Indicates the clinical utility of the test

– Helps reconstruct the patient's clinical history

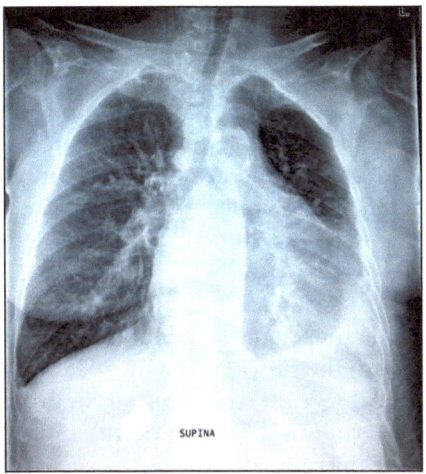

Fig. 49. Thorax X-ray. Pathological results must be described following a clinical hierarchy on the basis of their importance in connection with the patient's clinical picture. In this X-ray of the thorax, requested for control over congestive heart failure in a bedridden elderly patient, it would be better to describe first the signs of pulmonary congestion and then consider the nodular lesion present at the base of the left lung

the radiologist sees, but in all cases always using clinical common sense (Fig. 49) (see the chapter "Common Sense in Clinical and Preclinical Diagnosis").

Diagnostic Conclusion

This must briefly indicate the diagnostic interpretation given by the radiologist to the reports found, in both negative and positive cases. In the latter, it should be open and provide possibilities, as it is appreciated by the prescribing clinician who must draw an accurate diagnostic conclusion. When, however, it is not univocal, the radiologist should not indicate more than two hypotheses so as not to create confusion or mistrust in the prescriber.

Recommendation of Future Diagnostic Exams

Such recommendations must be made only if considered necessary. Otherwise, the radiologist risks becoming one of the main exam prescribers and cost generators, running the risk of not being believed and projecting an image of insecurity and uncertainty, which is not appreciated (Fig. 12) – just as with the too open or doubtful diagnostic conclusion mentioned above.

FOLLOW-UP EXAM

This is based on comparison with a previous exam – with the images and also with the report – because it is a subjective interpretation of images by a radiologist and, as such, is open to discussion. Therefore, the radiologist must be able to read the previous report well – that is, understand its clinical meaning and any limits or insufficiencies – while remaining in the sphere of a correct ethical sense (Figs. 30, 32).

ADDITIONAL EXAM

This must clarify the elements that remained doubtful or uncertain (Fig. 24) either because the previous diagnostic exam did not fully satisfy the clinical request or because it, in turn, raised perplexity or new uncertainties. Therefore, the report must be conclusive; otherwise the radiologist could be accused of poor efficiency. It must focus attention on the suspended diagnostic suspicion and mention the technique of execution used or chosen to solve it. All the rest is superfluous.

Chapter 13
Normality Reports Depending on the Subject's Age

Patient age can affect both the way the report is drawn up and the vocabulary used, especially as regards radiological reports that modify over the years or anatomical reports that, from time to time, become the reference according to age. This especially applies to children and the elderly, taken for granted that the reference model is that of adults.

A perfect example is the chest (Fig. 50). In children, the most specific anatomical reports are the pulmonary circle and the cardiovascular silhouette – vital for characterizing congenital defects (Fig. 51a) – and the pulmonary parenchyma in congenital and acquired phlogistic forms. In adults, such reports concern parenchyma in the research of focal, phlogistic, or neoplastic lesions; in elderly people, they concern the pulmonary circle and cardiovascular silhouette, as cardiac decompensation in its various stages is a prevailing pathology.

It is evident that if these clinical-anatomical targets are valid, the report cannot always be drawn up in the same way, especially in the sphere of normality. Therefore, in the radiological exam of the adult thorax, it is more important to look for focal parenchymal lesions, as the problems connected with bronchogenic neoplasia are prevailing. In the elderly, the state of the pulmonary circle should also be reported on, as problems connected with cardiac insufficiency are more important in such cases. It should also be remembered that the initial stages of cardiac insufficiency up to the interstitial edema may not be found during a physical exam, for which reason only the radiologist is able to give the correct diagnostic guidelines.

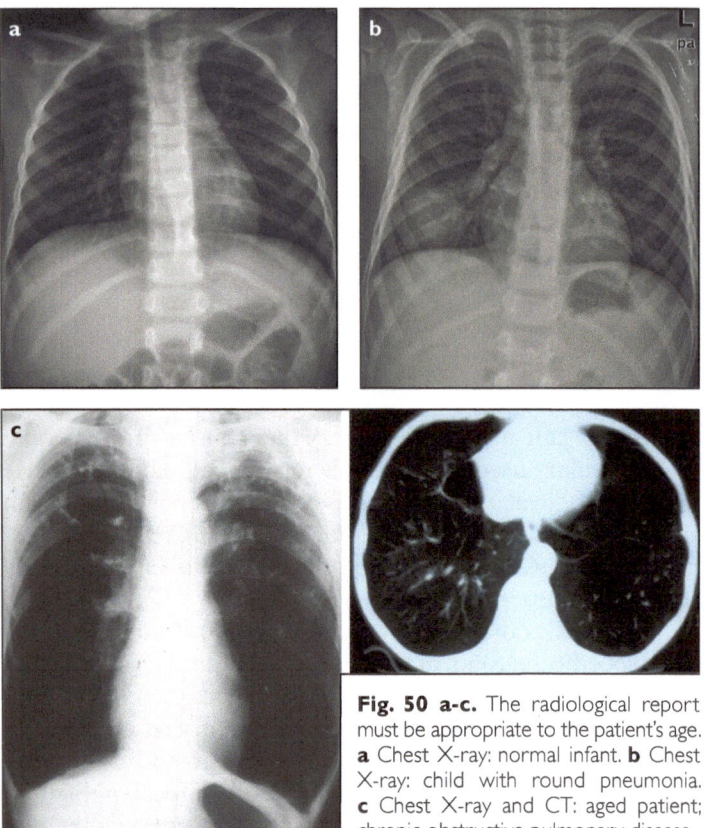

Fig. 50 a-c. The radiological report must be appropriate to the patient's age. **a** Chest X-ray: normal infant. **b** Chest X-ray: child with round pneumonia. **c** Chest X-ray and CT: aged patient; chronic obstructive pulmonary disease

Of course, focal parenchymal lesions also may be found in elderly people, but if there are also signs of cardiac decompensation, they must be highlighted and indicated first in the report, as they require immediate treatment (Fig. 49). Therefore, returning to a more general evaluation, normality should be reported in differentiated ways depending on age, and because each of us has our own individuality and guards it jealously.

Likewise, normality in children, if not recognized, can generate reports that are borderline cases to say the least, if not presumed pathologies (Fig. 51). As regards the cranium, we must consider the marked variability in dimensions, shape, thickness, and mineral content; the appearance of the diploic

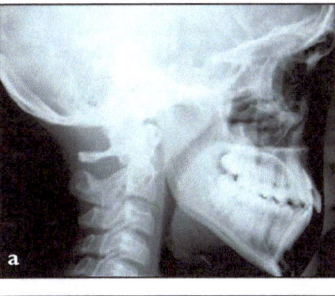
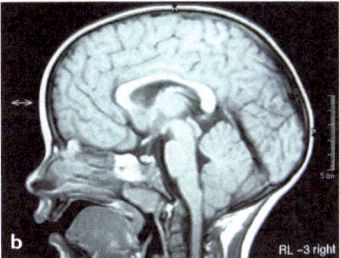
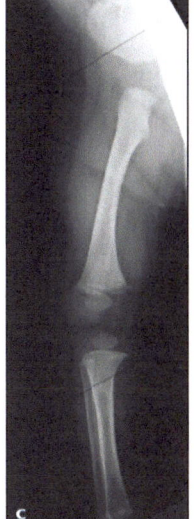

Fig. 51 a-c. Results considered normal changes according to patient age. **a** Aspect of the cranial base in a child (X-ray). **b** Encephalic ventricular system in a child (magnetic resonance). **c** Femur of a child (X-ray)

structure, dural sinuses, internal grooves, and vessels; the development of pneumatization of the temporal bones and the maxilla-facial bones; and the dimensions of form of the sella turcica. As regards the encephalon, variability in the amplitude of the ventricular system and the development of the corpus callosum must be considered, as when an MR exam is requested for a clinical suspicion of psychomotor deficiency. Concerning the pelvis, differences in the development and seat of the femoral cephalic nuclei must be considered, as in hip dysplasia screening if the objective exam is inconclusive.

In elderly people, the concept of normality is complicated with the distinction between normal and within the norm. Normal is what all elderly people have, such as long-sightedness; within the norm is what can be found in many subjects – but not all – according to a known and acceptable level, such as arthrosis. We must also bear in mind that the norm varies according to the socioenvironmental and cultural context. Therefore, atherosclerosis is within the norm for elderly people in industrialized countries but not for those in poor countries.

The above shows that there are many ways of confusing normal with pathological in elderly people (Fig. 52). The most

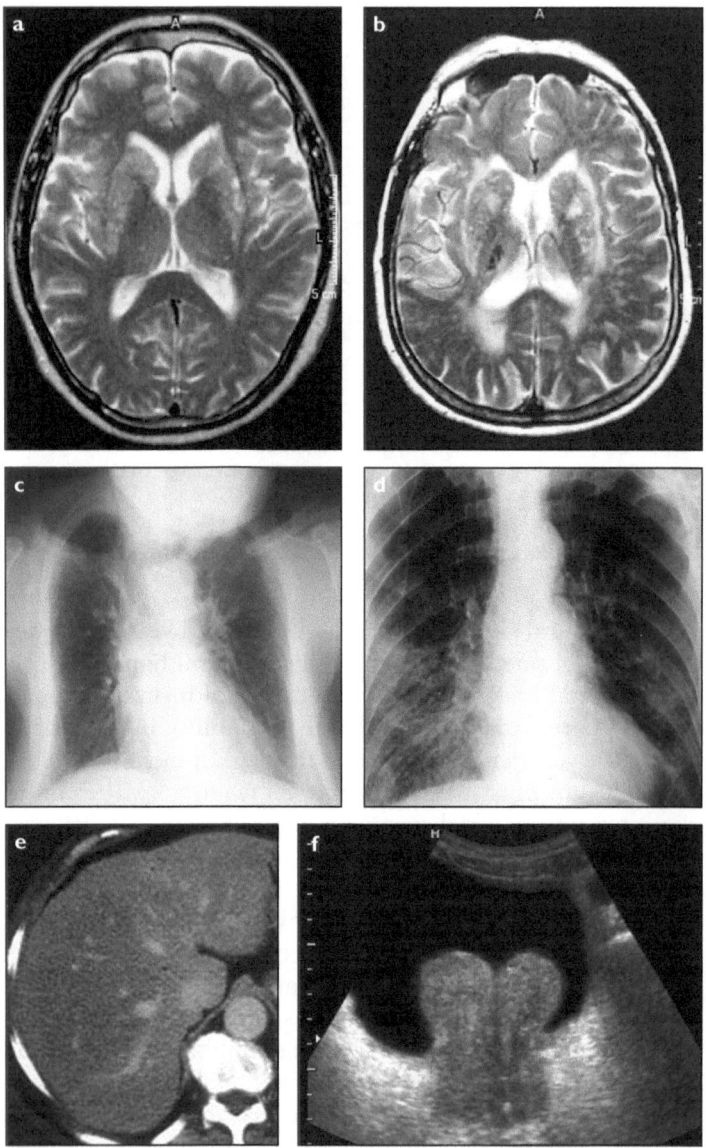

Fig. 52 a-f. In an elderly person, the border between physiological and para-physiological ageing can be quite shaded. **a** Brain physiological ageing [magnetic resonance (MR)]. **b** Chronic brain vasculopathy (MR). **c** "Cardiac lung" pattern (X-ray). **d** "Dirty" thorax pattern (X-ray). **e** Hepatic steatosis (computed tomography). **f** Benign prostatic hypertrophy (echography)

frequent are aspects of physiological cerebral ageing and signs of chronic vascular disease; signs of compatible osteoarticular involution and of pathology on a degenerative basis, such as indirect signs of shoulder rotator cuff tear due to impingement; the cardiac lung, as mentioned above, and the dirty thorax for visibility of bronchial pattern, possible expression of clinically latent chronic obstructive bronchopneumonia; the report of hepatic steatosis, visible both on the ultrasound and on the CT, more or less routine in elderly people but also a precocious sign of hepatopathy; dimensions and morphology of the prostate via a suprapubic ultrasound scan in an elderly person with latent clinical signs of hypertrophy.

These are all situations lying at the base of a simple question that is fundamental in geriatrics: Do we understand the ageing process, and at what point does physiology end and pathology begin?

Chapter 14
Errors in Reporting

Given that the report is a "professional" document and bears the associated responsibilities (as discussed in the chapter "Medical-Legal Aspects"), all of the radiologist's errors appear in it, either directly or indirectly. It is not easy to distinguish and classify the mistakes made when a report is prepared because, in most cases, the errors are complex and attributable to more than one cause and because many errors depend on the individual radiologist's professional, behavioral, and psychological traits. In fact, assuming that "anyone can make a mistake", some radiologists will make more mistakes than others because they are more predisposed to doing so (only those who are not paying attention make mistakes, as said in the "Introduction"), for which reason there are "universal" errors and "individual" errors: the first are committed by all radiologists; the second are not. These mistakes vary greatly (it suffices to think of those made due to a lack of respect for the logical sequence), but classifying them in this way could be too arbitrary. So, we have nothing more to say in that regard.

First, however, before going on, it is worth pointing out here a particular type of radiologist, one not included in the chapters on the reporter's sensitivity and psychological makeup, because it lies outside that context: the radiologist à la Forrest Gump. This is a superficial radiologist who generally does not ask questions and therefore finds no answers, who does not feel the need to examine issues in depth because he or she is convinced that his or her experience is sufficient and therefore does not question, and who – being essentially a simple, ingenuous person who acts in good faith – is not aware of his her professional limitations. A typical example is that given in Figure 53.

This having been said, mistakes may be divided into two major categories: perceptive and cognitive. They are all made within the framework of the image diagnostics system in which the radiologist works and with which he or she inter-acts. It is therefore possible to say that, in addition to the radiologist's own errors (the human errors discussed previously), there are systemic errors he or she inherits as the last player in the diagnostic procedure.

These two major categories are distinguished because the report is the result of a *perceptive* process and a *cognitive* process – very often interdependent – and is formulated with three different expressive procedures: (1) descriptive, con-nected to the concept of loyalty, as a result of which the better the description, the closer to the original – that is, to the doc-ument; (2) interpretive, subject to the concept of truth, be-cause it is limited and aimed at diagnosis definition and therefore verifiable; (3) decision-related, deriving from what is seen and interpreted.

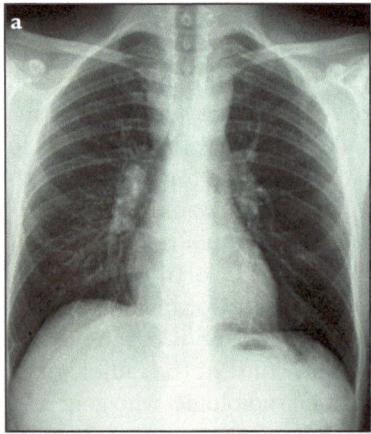

No evidence of pleuroparenchymatous lesions in active stage. Costophrenic sinuses free. Upper mediastinum bilaterally slightly enlarged. Heart image size within standard limits.

Fig. 53 a, b. X-ray of the thorax (**a**) and report (**b**). Reporting error owing to su-perficiality, that is, unwillingness to explore the case in depth to interpret the exhibits correctly. This is a case of sarcoidosis with three characteristic elements: mediastinum widening, hila enlargement, and pulmonary interstitial thread accentuation

The perceptive process is not a mere viewing but rather an extraction of images and their transformation into conscious assessment by means of the simplification and organization of peripheral information, that is, from the retina: what is perceived is thus not necessarily reliable and hence a first source of error.

The cognitive process is much more complex because it activates a broad mental field with ill-defined margins. It is therefore of use, in order to simplify, to refer to the Raufaste model, as applied to radiology (Fig. 54). It introduces the concept of dialogue between two memories: long-term, autonomous memory (and hence unconscious), with enormous possibilities for storage and containing theoretical and practical knowledge, the "nodes" connected to logical patterns (the "arches"); the other is working memory and depends on at-

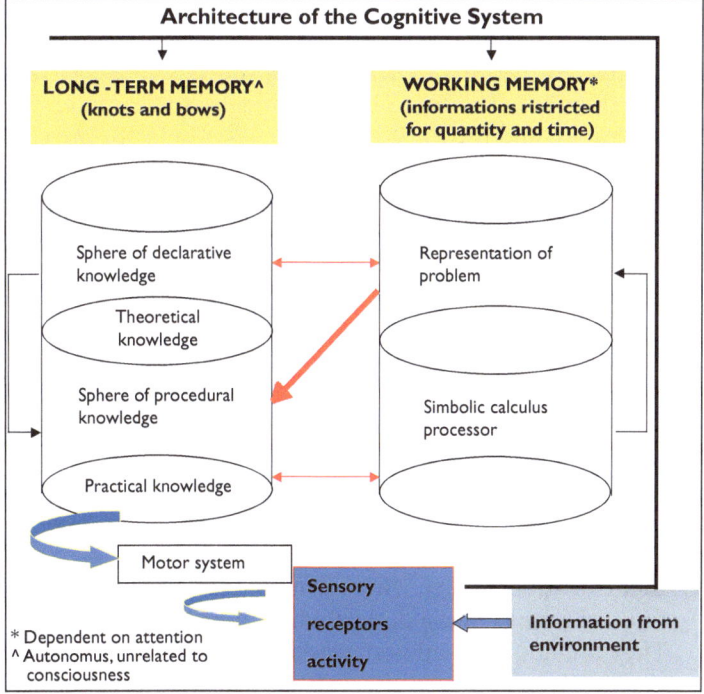

Fig. 54. Architecture of the cognitive system

tention, with the role of a symbolic calculating processor and of problem representation. The cognitive process as described is initiated by information collected from the environment by means of the sensory receptors and transmitted to the working memory, which calculates it symbolically and formulates the problem. It is then passed on to the long-term memory, which compares it with technical and practical knowledge and is included in a system that recalculates and recirculates it. This model makes the importance of *attention* very clear. Attention becomes a determining factor in professional activity and subsequent errors.

The professional activity is essentially based on three cognitive levels, which require an increasing degree of attention: (1) intellectual ability (skill), governed by defined patterns and models, for which the radiological signs lead directly to diagnosis; (2) rules (cognitive-ruled method), that require a model (for example, the presence of Kerley lines and/or a small, accentuated circle draws attention to a possible cardiomegaly and vice versa); and (3) knowledge, applied to new, unexpected situations that require an adjusted approach and deeper reasoning (Fig. 55). The first of these models is automatic, the second rapid, and the third long – the latter being at the root of so-called psychological errors.

Mistakes, as said before, are both perceptive and cognitive, and both in turn result in two major types of error: false positives and false negatives. Systemic or latent errors – also mentioned earlier – are a different situation and do not have an impact on the report.

Perceptive errors may involve nonidentification or erroneously attributed identification, whereas cognitive errors include oversights (skill errors) and those based on the cognitive or knowledge-based method, the so-called psychological errors (Fig. 56). All of these mistakes and the connections between them are summarized in the diagram given in Table 5. The different types of errors are now defined:

1. Identification errors with erroneous attribution: These types of errors consist of the finding of nonexistent lesions. They are not frequent and arise particularly during emergencies (such as identification of a nonexistent foreign body) but also as a result of choice (for example, an osteo-

phyte mistaken for a pulmonary nodule). They are essentially a distortion of the real facts.

2. Nonidentification errors without specific cause: These types of errors are much more frequent. Nonidentification errors without specific cause, otherwise known as "miss errors," may derive from the fact that perception is neither precise nor accurate, a result of human limitation, and are strongly influenced by expectations (for example, psychological pressure acting in any way on the reporter,

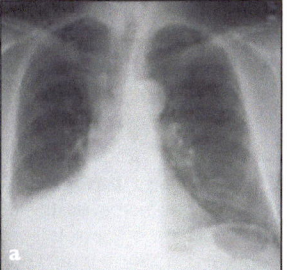

Fig. 55 a-c. The three levels of the cognitive process require increasing degrees of attention. Level 1: Activity based on the intellectual skill. This is ruled by predefined schemes and models (automatic); the radiological signs orientate directly toward the diagnosis, as in this case of lobar atelectasis (**a**, X-ray). Level 2: Activity based on rules (ruled cognitive method). This resembles the "if there is X, then Y…" model (fast); for example, small circle alterations draw attention to a possible cardiomegaly and vice versa (**b**, X-ray). Level 3: Activity based on knowledge. This is employed when facing new situations and demands reasoning and cultural adaptation (long); for example, the differential diagnosis between arachnoid and dermoid cyst (**c**, magnetic resonance)

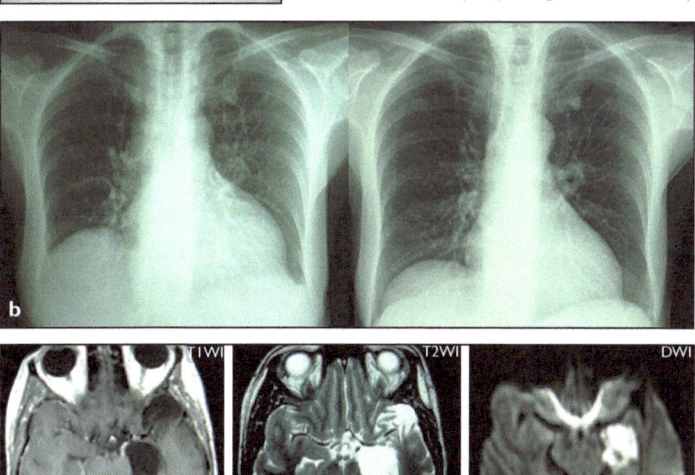

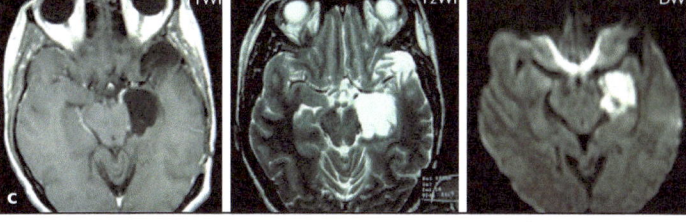

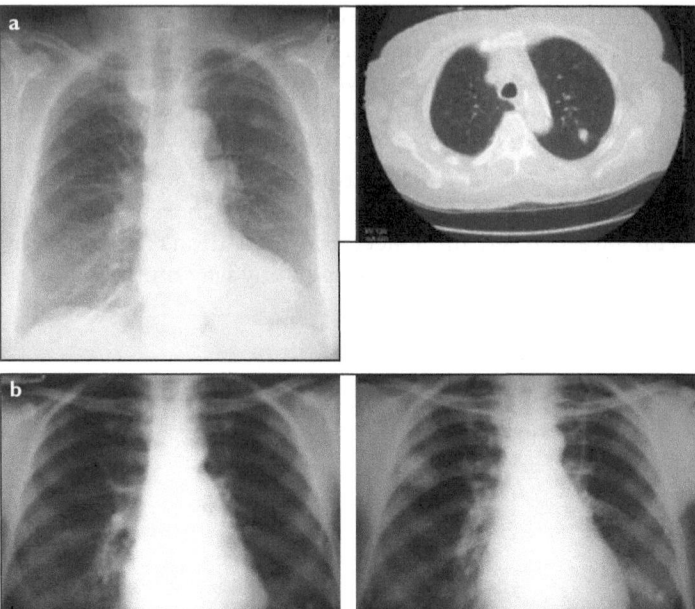

Fig. 56 a, b. Perceptive and cognitive errors. **a** Identification error with wrong attribution: pulmonary nodule mistaken for costal bone callus. **b** Underevaluation of the pathological exhibit: the right subclaviar pulmonary nodule is only pointed out but not appropriately described (no diagnostic in-depth examination is requested), so that at the next checkup, after 6 months, it has turned into "mass"

Table 5. Radiological Activity: Errors and Causes

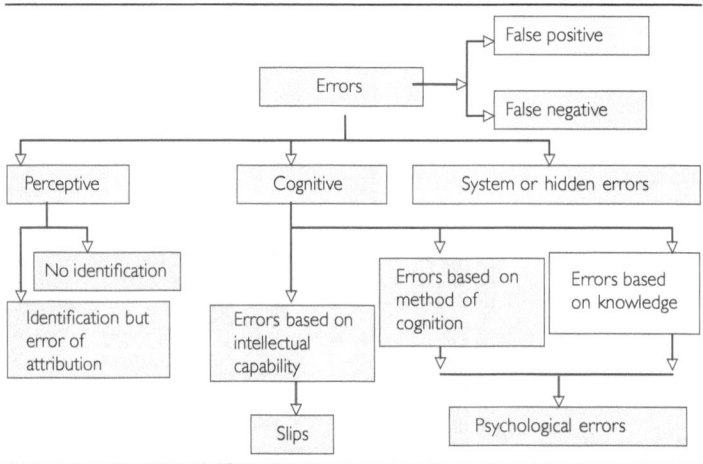

from the mere physical presence of the clinician to persistent requests, and may generate identification errors and even errors in writing). In many cases, it is a question of lesions that are easily recognizable a posteriori but that, unfortunately, are omitted in the report. It is difficult to explain how it was not possible to see what everyone was able to see later. They are very frequent relative to certain parts of the body, such as the breast and the lung. In the latter, according to some authors, nodular or mass tumors of dimensions from 19 to 40 mm are missed in 19% of cases; according to other authors, up to 50% are missed.

3. Errors of nonidentification or nonperception with specific cause: these types of errors can be subdivided into the following causal errors: (a) technical; (b) due to anomalies outside the area being examined; (c) resulting from incomplete knowledge; (d) resulting from search satisfaction (Table 6):

   a. Those with a technical cause, such as inadequate equipment, overexposure or incorrect exposure, incorrect positioning: In all these cases, when, that is, the examinations are of low quality or incomplete, the radiologist should refuse to issue the report, which could be incorrect. In any event, the radiologist should follow Berlin's advice (one of the most authoritative experts in the field, he provides written guidelines drawn up by his department on image quality and on the technical factors used) and indicate in the report any lack

Table 6. Causes of No Identification in Radiological Activity

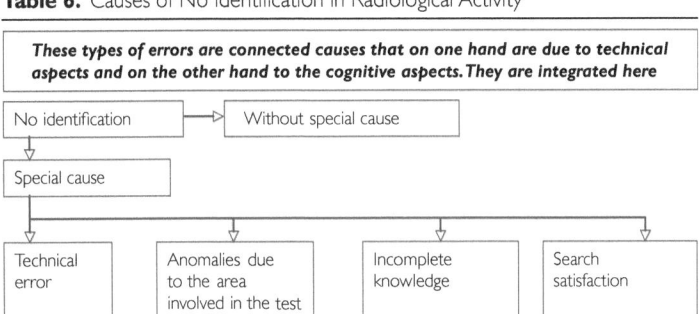

of quality or limitation with respect to the examination, and make a note of the impossibility of a certain interpretation when the patient is unavailable to have an examination repeated or completed.

b. Those with anomalies outside the area under examination: These errors occur when one area is being examined and no notice is taken of a visible lesion in another area (for example, a basal pulmonary lesion missed during a CT examination of the abdomen or, vice versa, an abdominal lesion missed during a thoracic examination or a pulmonary lesion missed during a back examination) (Fig. 57). These areas indicate the radiologist's lack of attention and are frequent when the report must be prepared in a hurry, such as during emergencies, and logically increase with the application of pan-explorative techniques.

c. Errors of incomplete knowledge: These result from ignorance, because what is not known is not seen and therefore does not appear in the report (the radiologist à la Forrest Gump). These errors have particularly to do with the lack of recognition of rarer anomalies or unusual situations (Fig. 58), with the lack of management of "borderline" lesions (Fig. 59), or insufficient application of new technologies and related semiotics; that is, in all situations that require greater knowledge.

d. Errors deriving from search satisfaction: These errors arise when once a significant lesion has been found and perhaps even answers the clinical question, the radiologist is satisfied, pays less attention, and does not perceive – thus omitting it from the report – another lesion that is potentially harmful to the patient (Fig. 60). But they can also arise during interpretation of mass examinations (such as in breast-cancer screening), when the discovery of a lesion reduces attention during subsequent examinations.

In all of these cases, the satisfaction gained from answering the pressing or particularly difficult clinical question – as in urgent or emergency situations – means that the rest is not recognized.

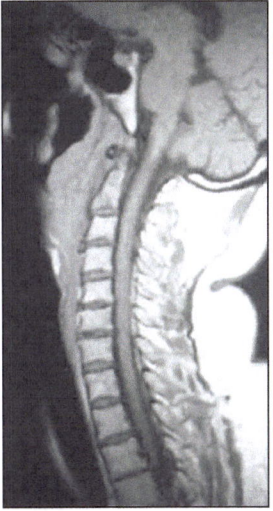

Fig. 57. Nonidentification error due to a specific cause (alteration out of the examination area). Focusing only on the anatomic region needed by the examination can lead to disregard for important pathological exhibits in adjacent regions. In this cervical column, magnetic resonance examination, requested for suspicion of discopathy, the radiologist focuses only on the cervical rachis, ruling out the presence of hernias, and so writes the report, without looking further. Thus, a lesion of the hypopharynx – that will prove to be neoplastic and which is the cause of the symptoms – escapes attention

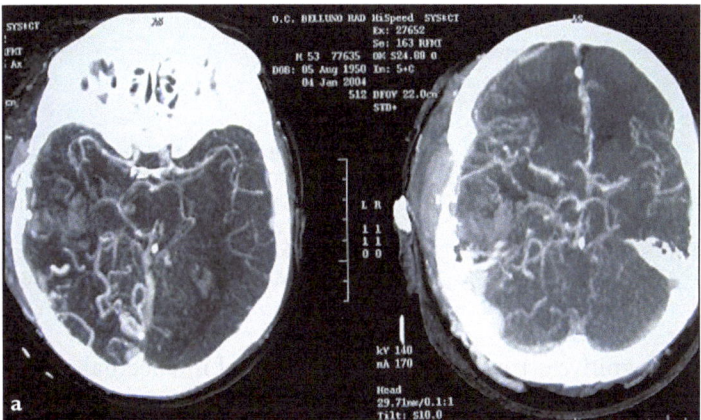

After-effects of a surgical operation in the right parietotemporal area with hemoventricle. ...
The angio-CT study of the Willis poligone points out an asymmetry of distribution of the vessels with increased caliper branch, with a winding course in the occipital area ascribable to the hypertrophy of the right posterior cerebral artery.

Fig. 58 a, b. Error owing to incomplete knowledge. The general radiologist generically and imprecisely describes a dural fistula because of lack of experience in the neuroradiological field

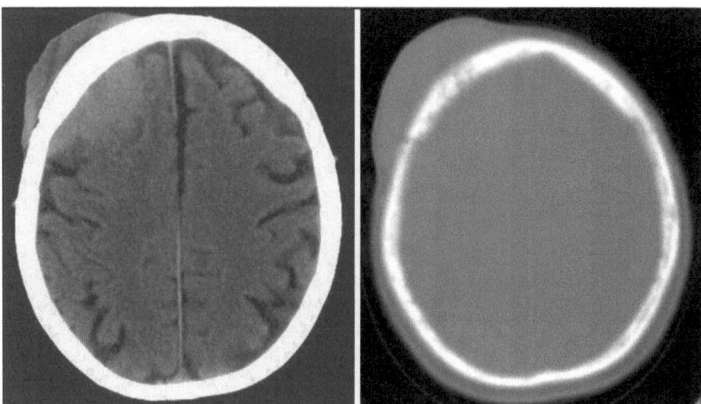

Fig. 59. Incorrect interpretation of an extracerebral lesion. Here the patient is subjected to cerebral computed tomography for trauma: the radiologist interprets the pattern as a posttraumatic extra-axial hematoma, without considering the real morphodensitometry of the lesion or the cranial-wall osteolytic alterations (lymphoma of the cranial theca)

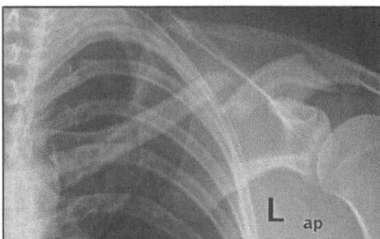

Fig. 60. Error owing to satisfaction in the research. Recognition of the displaced distal middle-third clavicular fracture "distracted" the radiologist from recognizing the extreme distal clavicular fracture

4. Cognitive errors: These are the result of intellectual ability (and are hence skill-based) and are both more complex and just as frequent. They are manifest as oversights (slipups) when attention wanders or is interrupted during routine activity. They may be expressed variously as the overlapping of reports, the right action on the wrong subject, temporary amnesia, etc. These are all situations characterized by a momentary lapse of attention and may have different causes, such as fatigue, insomnia, frustration, anxiety, overwork, etc. These mistakes occur more often during routine work than during emergencies. They may be manifest as the use of incorrect semiotics (for example, describing an

echograph as a CT or vice versa), with the confusion of an anatomical region (for example, the right wrist confused with the left wrist, or the abdomen with the chest, or vice versa), or even with the confusion of patients (one patient's identifying data confused with that of another).

5. Psychological mistakes: These are subject to so-called "bias" and may be one of two types: (1) rule-based, that is, deriving from the assessment of a contingent condition with an erroneous procedure, and hence the lack of application of a rule (actual errors); (2) knowledge-based, that is, deriving from the application of inadequate knowledge (true mistakes). In other words, the first occur during practice; the second during the practice of science. Both are errors of awareness because they derive from a judgment that is considered to be correct. These psychological errors may be both recognition errors and decision errors. In most cases, they are concomitant. They may derive from various factors: the habit of reasoning in a certain way; the awareness of an error on immediately subsequent behavior; the influence of clinical/anamnestic information (as discussed in the chapter "Considerations on the Usefulness of the Clinical Description"), particularly on false positives (for example, in a 1992 study by Norman, the clinical diagnosis of bronchiolitis in children, later proven to be overestimated, caused a significant increase in radiological false positives).

6. Errors caused by the influence of the clinical context: These types of errors are inevitable and frequent and can be reduced to the radiologist's clinical knowledge. Thus, faced with pulmonary thickening in a child or an adult/elderly person, a diagnosis of simple bronchopulmonitis will be plausible in the first case but more insidious in the second.

7. The so-called alliterative mistake: This is a repetitive mistake, for example, if the preceding radiologist – and even more so if recognized as being reliable and highly skilled (see the chapter "The Psychology of a Good Report: Radiologist and User") – makes an error, it is very probable that the subsequent radiologist will make the same error (Fig. 33). Here, as well, Berlin's suggestions may be of use: comparison with the documentation but not with the report,

which is examined only at the end; critical comparison of reports, so as to acquire new clinical information or to propose alternative hypotheses in order to resolve discrepancies. This is an error prevalent among young, relatively inexpert, radiologists, who are more psychologically dependent and have a less highly developed critical sense.

Chapter 15
The Structured Report and PACS

The structured report presupposes evaluation of its two constituent elements: the digital report and diagnostic-image management, that is, management of the "native" images and/or of their processing.

1. Digital report: in Europe, the digital report is regulated by several codified regulations. For example we report Italian low 59/97 states: "Records, data and documents produced by the public administration and private parties by computerized means ... their electronic storage and transmission, are valid and relevant to all effects of the law..." and "In all computer documents, the manual signature is replaced by the digital signature". Legislative Decree 82/2005, Article 22, states: "Documents produced by computerized means, computerized data and documents produced by public administrations constitute primary and original information..." This means that the written and signed digital report is an original, unique document and that, if the radiologist writes two reports, they are two originals and all others are copies. The report, once validated and digitally signed, is available online and may be accessed and consulted only by those so authorized (the user, the family physician, the consultant).

2. Diagnostic-image management: There are at least a few aspects of diagnostic-image management that are connected to the structured report. Firstly, the technological/computerized evolution of image diagnostics, thanks particularly to multi-image procedures (such as multislice CT), This requires automated, computerized systems able to rapidly

transmit and make available to the radiologist, almost in real time, the necessary data and at the same time obliges the radiologist to transmit his or her own data rapidly and efficiently. Secondly, the introduction of new diagnostic elements – such as bidimensional and tridimensional processing and reconstruction or elements deriving from assisted diagnosis or virtual reality (Fig. 61) – that must be made part of the reporting process.

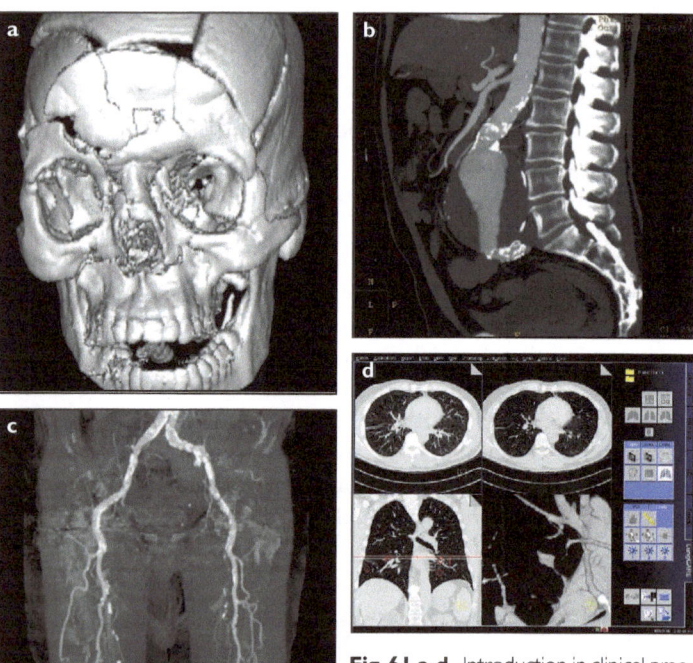

Fig. 61 a-d. Introduction in clinical practice of the system of elaboration in 2D and 3D digital images and the computer-assisted diagnosis (CAD) systems are rendering "insufficient" the traditional medical report – considered as text only – and opening the way for the "structured" medical report as the optimum tool to integrate the report with images. **a** Computed tomography (CT) of the splanchnocranium: 3D reconstruction. **b** CT angiography: maximum intensity projection (MIP) reconstruction of the abdominal aorta. **c** CT angiography: MIP reconstruction of the arteries of the lower limbs. **d** CAD system for study of pulmonary nodules

These very aspects also demonstrate the limits of the traditional report in the various phases of its preparation: image analysis, dictation, transcription, correction and signing, classification, fee payment, distribution, each one of which may be the source of mistakes. Limitations of the traditional report include the time required to produce and deliver the report; often incomplete formulation; unsatisfactory content; often unclear, if not actually ambiguous, language; insufficient standardization.

The digital report, as things stand today, is also limited because it may be available only as a simple text file or even stored as an archive file, which means that only in very few cases and at high cost can the information useful for scientific, teaching, administrative, and management purposes be extracted.

The structured report could be the tool that makes it possible to summarize and satisfactorily transmit the results of the radiologist's professional activity. This possibility has been discussed for many years, in fact as early as the 1960s. However, the principal projects actually carried out at the present time – the Missouri Automated Radiology System (MARS) and the Beth Israel Hospital Code Language Information Processing System (CLIP), have both had very restricted success because of a major limitation: the lack of a common vocabulary.

Subsequent efforts have therefore focused on this aspect, such as with the Radiological Society of North America (RSNA) initiative for a common vocabulary, known as Radlex and available on the Internet, and David Clunie's *DICOM Structured Reporting* manual. Clunie can be considered as the true inventor of the structured report to the extent that, today, the structured report is part of the digital imaging and communications in medicine (DICOM) standard.

But what actually is a structured report?

> **Top Tip!**
>
> A structured report is an electronic document in which the various parts of the report are qualified and structured, accompanied by the most significant images from among those assembled, in a standard format that can be used by health care computer systems.

A structured report is an electronic document that consists of all the parts considered as essential for a good report: patient's personal data; type of examination done; medical history; clinical request; examination's technical data; description of hierarchized reports and any measurements, accompanied by the images; diagnostic conclusions; coding for the pathology in question (Fig. 62).

In this case, the word "standard" should not be understood as a homogenization of the work or as the attempt to impose a leveling out of reporting according to preestablished models but, rather, as the possibility to distribute the report widely and to process it and maintain a history of it for an indefinite period of time, thanks to computer technologies.

Its principal advantages are its completeness because, in addition to what has already been said, it may also include other multimedia elements, such as audio, video, etc; the speed with which it can be produced; its legibility and clarity; the possibility of comparison with subsequent checks; and format standardization.

But the structured report also offers other possibilities, such as templates, which enable assisted reporting, as in the event of the description of a lesion when the radiologist may choose from a list the morphological characteristics that are closest to the description (Fig. 63). Templates also make it

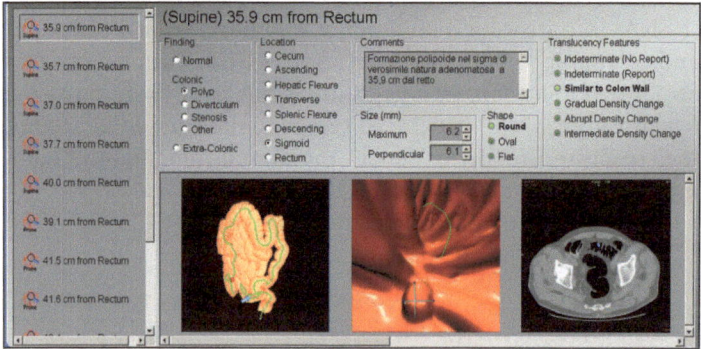

Fig. 62. The structured medical report is an informatics document in which the different parts of the report results are codified and structured, complete with the most significant images, through links in a standard format, which is made available by the databases of health systems

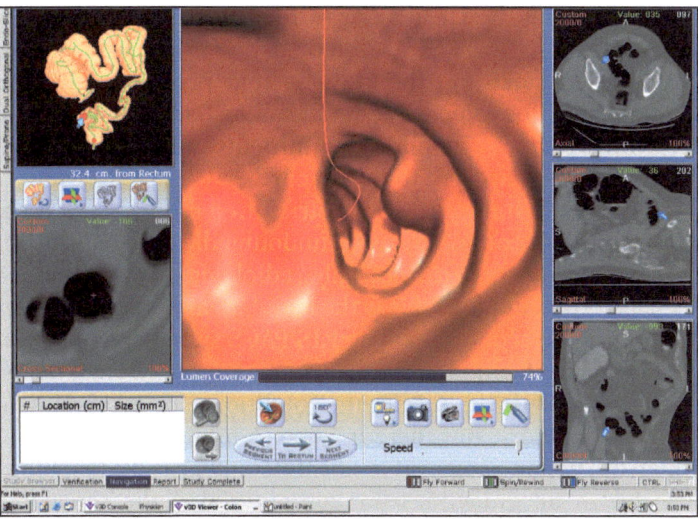

Fig. 63. The structured report enables assisted reporting. This may be in the description of a lesion when the radiologist may choose morphological characteristics from a list that are closest to his or description. Or it may make it possible to identify the most significant images for the purposes of interpreting and arriving at the diagnostic conclusions the radiologist has made. Or, finally, it makes use of consistent presentation of images, that is, the possibility of storing and "freezing" the processing of, and modifications to, the images evaluated, and of adding notes, to facilitate and focus comparison with images from subsequent examinations

possible to identify the most significant images for the purposes of interpreting and arriving at the diagnostic conclusions the radiologist has made, which are automatically noted and classified in the pre-report. Finally, they make use of consistent presentation of images, that is, the possibility of storing and "freezing" the processing of and modifications to the images evaluated and of adding notes so as to facilitate and focus comparison with the images from subsequent examinations. Another advantage of the structured report is that it means that delivering a CD to the patient with all the documentation produced becomes pointless, because a document is made available containing the most important images, while it remains possible to provided the entire documentation, such as in the case of oncological examinations. The report thus fulfills all specifications requested by the Integrating the Health Care Enterprise (IHE), a framework set out by the RSNA. The objective is to integrate the structured report and the systems that produce it within modern radiology departments and that harmonize it with electronic-folder systems, the imminent future of information technology applied to health care.

However, in Italy at least, the structured report is still little known and not commonly used, undoubtedly due to a lack of knowledge that concerns not only radiologists but the industry itself. An example of this is the fact that, as part of a call for tenders for the acquisition of an RIS/PACS system, compliance with IHE specifications is neither requested nor offered, nor is compliance with the minimum conditions for producing a structured report. But there is hope. A joint round table, in which the Italian Society of Medical Radiologists participated, has drawn up guidelines for computerizing the reporting process, and these guidelines are about to be published. The radiologist's qualifying contribution is identified in these guidelines with the production of the structured report. When the document has been published, it will also have official, regulatory weight.

The structured report cannot, however, be considered as a panacea that will solve all the current problems and limits of reporting. On the other hand, it may be the best solution for creating the homogeneous report so hoped for by physicians. It may also be the most effective means of arriving at medical-legal protection for radiologists, insofar as the images chosen and included by the radiologist become the "proof" of diagnostic accuracy.

PACS increases the radiologist's autonomy. The radiologist becomes the direct manager of all report-production phases, able to correct it and modify it in real time while analyzing the images. In this way, it undoubtedly improves report quality, although it does require a certain degree of learning and, in general, additional time is required for management of the computer system used. The most valuable use of the structured report depends on optimization of the working method and integration of computer systems through application of the IHE protocol.

Chapter 16
Radiological Reporting in the United States

Radiologists in the United States are voluminous producers and a major contributor to the US $6- to 12-billion transcription industry. The volume and complexity is constantly increasing, as is the number of images for review. In a recent review, Rick Marin at the Mayo Clinic, Jacksonville, FL, USA, tracked the number of computed tomography (CT) images produced in the department and compared this to prior years (Table 7).

Ongoing developments and advancement of integrated imaging, higher resolution scans, and more slices means that this problem is set to increase. By James Thrall's estimates from the Massachusetts General Hospital in Boston, MA, USA, we can expect at least a 50% increase in imaging volume in the next 5 years.

With that in mind, and with the constant changes in images to be reported on and the increasing pressure on time, American radiologists are under increasing stress to produce their report quickly and consistently. For many, the challenge is keeping up with the workload and remaining current with latest practices and innovations. Over the course of the last

Table 7. Comparison of Images Produced and Read in 2002 and 2006

Year	Number of CT image Images/day	Time to read per image (s/image)
2002	16,000	2
2006	80,000	0,45

few years, there has been a dramatic and significant shift toward electronic documentation and the introduction of speech recognition – a tool that has not been without problems historically but has truly reached tipping point for implementation in radiology practices today. The premature introduction of the technology and unrealistic expectations certainly hindered – and probably delayed – acceptance of the technology. Very early implementation of speech recognition was inevitably limited due to the requirement for pauses between the dictation of each report. However, with the introduction of continuous speech recognition in 1993, at the Radiological Society of North America (RSNA), radiologists became one step closer to the future that Hollywood had been selling for the previous 20 years – talking to computers would be the best method of interacting with technology. Sadly, this introduction concealed the significant hardware inadequacies of the day, and whereas it was possible to achieve good results, it required an uneconomical investment in information technology and too much effort on the part of a busy radiologist.

Fast forward 14 years, and hardware brings increasingly effective performance at lower prices. Also, refinement of the engine has put speech recognition front and center in the radiologists' armory, helping them achieve higher productivity and greater efficiency while satisfying the instant reporting requirements that are increasingly necessary in the delivery of high-quality care.

There is another significant pressure on radiologists in the United States – the need for rapid communication is well documented and necessary to improve quality of care; however, there is also the competitive pressure to match service levels of other radiologist in the surrounding area. So, if the local private radiology center is offering a 2-h report turnaround time, then to compete for that business and continue to be successful in what is a competitive market, the local radiologists have to deliver the same level of service. This is an ongoing process and will continue to improve service levels. To meet that need, radiologists must continue to innovate in their methods and offer better service, which represents an ongoing challenge with the other pressures of increasing volume of complexity and number of images that need to be reviewed.

Efficiency becomes a major driver for radiologists, and anything that allows them to achieve higher throughput and deliver more reports in less time is a welcome tool. Speech recognition has certainly helped drive some of the efficiencies that radiologists now enjoy, but there are some side benefits to this tool that provide time and cost savings. Historically, radiologists would gather routine reports and provide these to their secretary or transcriptionists who would store these "canned" or standard reports. These reports would then be accessed by the individual physician or sometimes a group of physicians who would dictate a few words to trigger the use of a template or standard report. For example: "normal chest X-ray". These three words might generate a three-section report for a normal chest X-ray and would typically be accessed by the transcriptionist with a few simple keystrokes. The value of this was in time savings, for both the radiologists and the transcriptionist. The method was refined over time and became more sophisticated with the addition of fields that could be customized as part of the dictation, thereby including specific data that was linked to that film and that patient.

This concept of standard or canned reports generates responses that are negative and positive. On the positive end, there is consistency in reports and information capture and presentation, and a saving in time and resources to report on normal images. On the negative side, there is a view that it can increase the opportunity for radiologists to miss significant clinical findings, as the provision of standard text might decrease the use of a rigorous methodology of review of an image and the process of reporting on that image. In addition, there are some that view the process of dictating as part of the review process, forcing the radiologist to step through the systematic review of an image, a process that aids in ensuring that findings are not missed. There are also those who consider this cheating, as the radiologist is paid to review the image, and using a "canned" report does not actually provide a customized review of that image. However, in this instance, the benefits outweigh the drawbacks, and although there are detractors, the use of standard "canned" reports is prevalent in radiology and deemed acceptable, not least of all given the significant skew of normal (8% or more) to abnormal reports (20% or less).

Diagnostic radiology is a very fast-paced profession. A private-practice diagnostic radiologist will read anywhere from 60 to 160 exams in a day, with the number of exams depending on multiple variables, including whether the practice is centered in a hospital or an imaging center and whether it is based in an academic institution or is a purely private practice. Radiologists have moved away from the view stations in front of radiographic light boxes or rotating light boxes – called "rotor viewers" – to digital viewing stations. The rooms are generally dark, and the radiologist has a dictation system, although increasingly, the dictation system and transcription is being replaced by real-time speech-recognition systems that render the report immediately for signature and distribution. The diagnostic radiologist reads the film and dictates his or her findings, impression and differential diagnosis.

Much of the fast pace stems from the fact that as the radiologist is reading his or her studies, there are frequent interruptions from multiple sources, including referring physicians asking about particular patients, technologists asking about technical details of studies they are performing, and staff interrupting for a multitude of reasons. This breaks the radiologist's train of thought and can make it difficult and frustrating to keep up with the number of exams that must be read that day. The work day is normally well defined, and excess work load is either read by all the radiologists until everything is complete or in some cases, a group may designate one or more radiologists to stay until to do "cleanup" of any outstanding images that require reporting. Radiologists also work on call, and this also used to require attending the hospital or practice to view images. Increasingly, however, the images can be sent externally to radiologists in their homes to view and report remotely: teleradiology. In some cases, the out-of-hours work is outsourced to a service that provides cover for this purpose. These services are often referred to as "nighthawks". Depending on the group, the nighthawks may come from within the group or the call may be outsourced. In academic practices, the call is usually performed by the residents at the academic center.

Reporting process and style varies widely throughout the United States and is driven by factors that might not impact reporting in other countries. Market forces and demand are at work here, and these shape the different methods, tools, and processes. Even location and geography have been significant drivers of methods and styles, with different approaches to reporting in an academic institution where in many cases the medical staff is employed and answerable to the hospital versus the small radiology clinics or service with no radiologists on staff.

In broad terms, radiologists are interactive with the departments in which they work, although for many of the plain films and simple studies, the radiologist's actual involvement in image acquisition is limited or nonexistent. This shift is well demonstrated by the increase in successful teleradiology services that report on films that originate in another state or even country, but it does come with challenges associated with reporting on images from other states (see section "Remote Reporting Issues: Credentialing and State Licensure").

Many radiologists working in groups focus on a specific room or image type for a set period of time, typically a morning or afternoon but perhaps a smaller segment of time. In most cases, automated systems allocate the images for reporting based on this segregation of images.

This process does typically require some level of automation and a move toward electronic environments with radiology information systems (RIS) and picture archiving and communication systems (PACS). Even in traditional plain-film departments, this segregation of work still occurs but is harder to achieve. With the advent of RIS management systems that automate much of the workflow and the transmission of information between the various team members in a radiology department, it is possible to segregate and subspecialize image reporting. And whereas many radiologists report on more than one area and on other images, many focus on a specific area of imaging and subspecialty. Digital systems allow clinical information and images to flow to radiologists in any location and to group studies by procedure and area of specialization. The digital automation also speeds the process of presenting the images to the radiologists by removing the need for the manual process of printing and hanging the films ready for reading by radiologists. A residual benefit of this is the inbuilt flexibility of the hanging protocols built into digital systems that allows for the same reading station to be used by many radiologists. It also removes the need for technologists and support staff to memorize different reading requirements of individual radiologists, as the technology takes care of these factors automatically. The additional removal of the lag time for the image to reach the radiologists means that reporting can commence much earlier, thereby decreasing further the time from study to report.

Radiologists are allocated images and sit in a customized area that has been optimized for reading. In most cases, this customization might be standard for all rooms, but in recent months, several institutions have started to experiment with varied reporting environments (see HealthImaging.com: Chesson, Erin, "Reading Room Essentials", December 1, 2006; http://www.healthimaging.com/content/view/5425/110/). However, these innovations are yet to hit mainstream radiology reporting environments.

Historically, reporting was a dictation-based activity that found the radiologist reviewing images on a light box and dictating into a microphone and a tape-based recording device. This audio recording would be carried to the transcriptionist who would have to be physically located nearby to receive the tape. The report would be transcribed and returned in printed form for review. Any changes would need to be manually applied and returned to the transcriptionists for correction and resubmission. Once the report was correct, the radiologists would sign it and it would be distributed to referring physicians and filed in the medical report. The process was inefficient but provided a typed and legible report that could be used for clinical care and provided the basis for billing the insurance company or other payer for the radiologist's reporting services.

Innovation to this method included the introduction of digital-telephony-based dictation that utilized the telephone as the input device and recorded the dictation on a computer either locally or centrally located but connected to the telephone system. This provided some significant flexibility in the transmission of the audio report to the transcriptionists, who could then be positioned in any location that had access to a telephone. This innovation led to the move of the transcriptionist away from individual departments to pools centrally located and was a major contributor to the boom in the out-sourced transcription marketplace that exists in the United States today. There still remain transcriptionists tied to departments and individual radiologists and even continued usage of audiotapes to transmit the audio report, but this practice is increasingly being replaced by the more flexible digital recording.

Capture of audio into a digital form provided the opportunity to innovate and introduce speech recognition technology, and today, more than 15% of radiology practices (see *Radiology Today*: Roop, Elizabeth S. "Sorting Out Speech Recognition", June 19, 2006, 7(12)18; http://www.radiologytoday.net/archive/rt06192006p18.shtml) is using speech recognition, and in some cases, 100% of a radiology department or facility is using speech recognition to support their reporting activity. There are many forms and different implementations of this technology (see section "Speech Recognition Technology"), but the solution is similar throughout. Audio dictated by the radiologists is captured and converted into a digital sound file. That digital sound file is processed by the engine, which produces its best interpretation of the audio converted into words.

Typically, radiologists process images in accordance with a systematic and structured sequence, reviewing films to identify air, fat, soft tissue, bone, and in some cases metal and contrast agents. This section cannot cover the full details of this process, and the reader can find many extensive books and articles on the systematic process of reviewing radiographic images. For the purposes of this chapter, the discussion is limited to the general process and system to provide some insight. Some advocate a free search pattern either as the initial approach to the film, which is then followed by an organized search if some abnormality is found, or as the final scan of an apparently normal film. Most experienced radiologists interpret films in this manner (Tuddenham WJ, Culvert WP. Visual search patterns in roentgen diagnosis. *Radiology* 1961;76:255–256; Tuddenham WJ. The visual physiology of roentgen diagnosis. A. Basic concepts. *Am J Roentgenol* 1957;78:116–123). However, the formalized approach, which varies by film type and imaging modality, can be summarized as follows:

Technical Quality

- Is the film correctly centered?
- Is the patient rotated?
- Does the film include all areas?
- In the cases of moving areas, are they in the right phase (for example, full inspiration)?
- Is the exposure correct?

Symmetry

- Film should be symmetrical where appropriate.

Soft Tissue

- Typically, working either from the outside peripheral tissue in or vice versa, looking for any increase, decrease, absence, or asymmetry, of soft tissue. Evidence of air, either appropriate or inappropriate, and its distribution.

Osseous Structures

- View the osseous structures and trace outlines of all areas looking for lack of continuity; demineralization; joints.

Other Areas

- In the case of a plain film of the chest, the review should also include specific areas such as the mediastinum and surrounding structures, hilum, heart, and the great vessels, including size and position, and the lung fields.

The report produced by radiologists almost always follow the same sequence, with some variation by imaging modality and anatomical location, it but consists of these main areas:

- Procedure or examination description
- Clinical information (if available)
- Technique (if applicable)
- Comparisons (if any)
- Findings
- Impression

Each section will vary in content and size depending on the actual image being reported on. For example, the Procedure may be absent or very limited in the case of a plain-film chest X-ray versus a contrast-enhanced computed tomography (CT) scan of the abdomen. In some cases with the use of clinical systems, some of this information is captured automatically and may be transmitted from the technologist (for example, the procedure details may be captured by the radiology technician).

In many cases, the radiology technician also captures clinical details, although the transmission of this information has not been well handled to date in the paper-based system. With the increasing connectivity of systems and the automated transmission of clinical data, radiologists are now finding they have access to many more clinical details than they did historically that relate to the image they are reading. This provides added advantage to help in the accurate reading of images.

SPEECH RECOGNITION TECHNOLOGY

The process of speech recognition requires that sound be converted from a recording of our voice via a microphone (an analog signal) into digital chunks of data that the computer can analyze. It is from this data that the computer must extract enough information to confidently predict the words being spoken. In simple terms, this digital data stream has the following steps applied to recognize the text contained in it:

Step 1: Extracting Phonemes

In the first step, phonemes are extracted – these are best described as sounds that group together to form our words.

Examples of Phonemes

aa	f<u>a</u>ther
ae	c<u>a</u>t
ah	c<u>u</u>t
ao	d<u>o</u>g
aw	f<u>ou</u>l
ng	si<u>ng</u>
t	<u>t</u>alk
th	<u>th</u>in
uh	b<u>oo</u>k
uw	t<u>oo</u>
zh	plea<u>s</u>ure

The English language uses about 40 phonemes to convey the 500,000 or so words it contains; other languages have different phonemes and word counts. Phonemes are often extracted by running the waveform through a Fourier transform.

Step 2: Converting Phonemes into Words and Sentences

The phonemes have to be converted into words and sentences. The most common method to achieve this uses a statistical analysis tool based on a concept called Hidden Markov Model (HMM) that makes the statistical probability analysis of the phonemes faster and more efficient. Differentiating between similar-sounding phonemes and producing the correct text is not as easy as one might think – for instance:

"Recognize speech"
"Wreck a nice beach"

These two phrases are surprisingly similar, yet have wildly different meanings. A program using a Markov Model at the sentence level might be able to ascertain which of these two phrases the speaker was actually using through statistical analysis using the phrase that preceded it.

In addition to the basic engine for recognizing words, most speech engines now include customization to the individual's speaking style, typical speaking content (grammar and vocabulary), and acoustic details of their speech pattern using a specific dictation device (for instance, a telephone, microphone, or hand-held digital recorder) – the acoustic reference file. The content produced then becomes the basis for the report, which is either edited by physicians themselves (so-called front-end speech recognition) or passed to a transcriptionist or medical editor who reviews the output, corrects any mistakes, and then returns it to the radiologists for approval and signature – so-called back-end speech recognition.

Experienced medical transcriptionists are highly efficient workers who have developed tools and techniques over time to improve productivity. Word expanders, shortcut keys, and, in some cases, speed-typing tools, increase their productivity to over 160 lines per hour. Presenting a speech recognition draft of the dictated report offers some efficiencies that are dependent on several factors:

- Accuracy of the draft: Higher accuracy results in increased productivity improvements. Retyping missed or grossly inaccurate text requires more time and effort and reduces the efficiency gains.
- Ease of correction of errors: Not all errors are created equal.
- Deleting superfluous text: Dictation may include, "This is Dr. van Terheyden dictating on patient Glenn Bow". If the software can automatically dictate information already in the report header or is otherwise superfluous, it can save the transcriptionist time.
  Minor corrections within the text are relatively easy.
- Correction tools and feedback to the medical transcriptionist/medical editor.
- Dictating style, pronunciation, and audio quality.

Front-end versus Back-end Speech Recognition

Back-end Speech Recognition
Physicians have typically been used to a back-end process in which the author dictates either by phone or into a handheld device and then passes this dictation on to transcriptionists for manual transcription. Back-end speech recognition applications copy this workflow and add speech recognition, enabling the transcriptionist to edit the automatically generated text instead of having to type the entire dictation. This workflow already significantly improved the process for both sides: doctors received reports more quickly, and transcriptionists were able to work more efficiently.

Pros for Back-end Speech Recognition
- Ideal for hospitals that do not want to involve physicians in the report transcription process.
- Doctors continue to work the same way as before (no change in behavior).
- Transcriptionists experience increased productivity.

Cons for Back-end Speech Recognition
- If corrected by transcriptionists, still makes doctors dependent on transcriptionists.
- Reports available after dictation, not during dictation.

- If interrupted, there is no immediate indication on screen where to continue dictation.

Front-end Speech Recognition

Front-end speech recognition gives physicians more flexibility and control, allowing them to create reports themselves without the involvement of a transcriptionist. Instead of having dictation recognized by the speech-recognition server in the background, the text is presented back to the physician in realtime, either while they dictate or immediately after they have completed dictation.

Pros for Front-end Speech Recognition
- Instant report production and availability.
- No delay in correction by clinicians – less likelihood of report errors.
- Auto text and templates available for more standardized, higher-quality reporting.

Cons for Front-end Speech Recognition
- May require some additional report creation time in the case of physician self-corrected documents.
- Requires some change in behavior of clinicians.

Intelligent Speech Interpretation

For years, speech recognition solutions have focused on the engine's accuracy, but in medical transcription, this does not tell the whole story. Even with a speech recognition rate of 100%, the document may still require significant adaptation and correction by the speaker or medical transcriptionist/editor. Typical medical reports are not actually dictated in the format of the final report. In addition, many speakers inject additional phrases and superfluous content that needs to be removed from the final report.

Medical transcriptionists therefore do much more than simply type what was dictated. First, they leave out the "ums" and "ers", ignore extraneous dialogue that does not belong in the dictation, automatically implement corrections that the doctor may or may not catch, fill information into forms, and even rephrase sentences. In addition, they format and organize the text by adding section headings, numbering lists, and including standard blocks of content. In short, they ensure that the final document communicates what the doctor meant, rather than just what he or she said.

Intelligent speech interpretation (ISI) (see section "Intelligent Speech Interpretation") emulates these capabilities in an effort to increase the transcription staff's productivity. ISI also includes punctuation assistance that eliminates the need for radiologists to dictate commas and periods.

Many radiologists dictate their reports as they are viewing the images, leaving large periods of silence. Transcriptionists used to waste a lot of time passing through these silences in the dictation. ISI automatically removes these pauses, providing a 30–50% percent in the time it takes to review radiology dictation.

REMOTE REPORTING ISSUES: CREDENTIALING AND STATE LICENSURE

The United States, while externally viewed as a single country, is really a federation of 51 countries with different rules and regulations and, more importantly, different medical credentialing requirements. To the external viewer, provision of service by a radiologist in New York to a patient imaged in California seems normal and easy to achieve with today's teleradiology concepts and tools. This, however, is not the case, and state laws impact the ability for companies to successfully deliver service across state lines. In fact, the complexity of this issue and the web of competing rules and regulations add an additional burden to the process and in many cases prevents the successful delivery of these services across state boundaries. In cases where this has been achieved it is typically with an added layer of workflow and management to ensure compliance with various state laws and regulations. A simple example of this is the routing of reports. For radiologists to be able to report on an image, they must be credentialed in that state and have a license to practice medicine in that state, as well as have radiology-board certification. In many cases, the process of obtaining that license and board certification makes it necessary for systems to track this information and use it as part of the image report assignment process. Urgency of images and availability and certification of individuals and their ability to report on images in other states must be taken into account. If an urgent case is imaged in Idaho and requires review but the available radiologists is not credentialed and licensed for that state, it is important that an alternative reader who is credentialed in Idaho can be found quickly to provide the required reading in a timely fashion.

Credentialing

Credentialing is one way hospitals can verify the quality of care being offered by their radiology staff. Done meaningfully, it gives the public confidence in the health care services and gives radiologists confidence they will only be asked to take responsibility for services for which they are appropriately skilled and experienced and that have been properly resourced. In many cases, a radiologist will be more broadly skilled than a particular post requires; by agreeing to the scope of practice for individuals, credentialing also ensures activity within any specialty that matches the department of radiology's current strategic plan and objectives. Credentialing thus allows both clinical staff and the hospital to be clear about what is expected and authorized.

Intelligent Speech Interpretation

To be beneficial for document creation, speech-recognition systems must be able to interpret what the speaker means, rather than just successfully recognize words. In part, this is because transcriptionists do much more than simply type what was dictated. For a start, they leave out the "ums" and "ehs", ignore dialogue that is not part of the dictation, implement corrections that are dictated as part of the text, enter information into forms, and even rephrase sentences. They format and organize text, adding section headings, numbering lists and standard blocks of content. In short, they ensure that the final document communicates what was meant, rather than just what was said. ISI technology emulates the capabilities of good medical transcriptionists to increase the productivity of secretarial staff and free resources for more critical tasks. Crucially, the technology is just as useful to doctors who prefer to look after the reporting process themselves as it is to those who delegate transcription and editing to someone else.

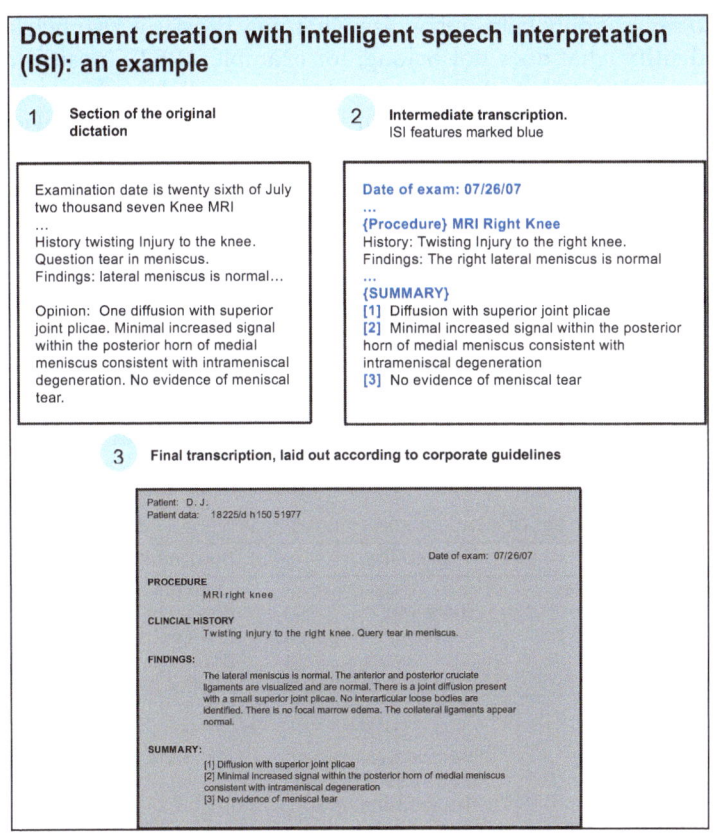

Document creation with intelligent speech interpretation (ISI): an example

1 Section of the original dictation

2 Intermediate transcription.
ISI features marked blue

Examination date is twenty sixth of July two thousand seven Knee MRI
...
History twisting Injury to the knee. Question tear in meniscus.
Findings: lateral meniscus is normal...

Opinion: One diffusion with superior joint plicae. Minimal increased signal within the posterior horn of medial meniscus consistent with intrameniscal degeneration. No evidence of meniscal tear.

Date of exam: 07/26/07
...
{Procedure} MRI Right Knee
History: Twisting Injury to the right knee.
Findings: The right lateral meniscus is normal
...
{SUMMARY}
[1] Diffusion with superior joint plicae
[2] Minimal increased signal within the posterior horn of medial meniscus consistent with intrameniscal degeneration
[3] No evidence of meniscal tear

3 Final transcription, laid out according to corporate guidelines

Patient: D. J.
Patient data: 18225/d h150 51977

Date of exam: 07/26/07

PROCEDURE
        MRI right knee

CLINICAL HISTORY
        Twisting injury to the right knee. Query tear in meniscus.

FINDINGS:
        The lateral meniscus is normal. The anterior and posterior cruciate ligaments are visualized and are normal. There is a joint diffusion present with a small superior joint plicae. No intrarticular loose bodies are identified. There is no focal marrow edema. The collateral ligaments appear normal.

SUMMARY:
        [1] Diffusion with superior joint plicae
        [2] Minimal increased signal within the posterior horn of medial meniscus consistent with intrameniscal degeneration
        [3] No evidence of meniscal tear

Situational Intelligence

The initial challenges in doing this are acoustics due to background noise, as well as differences in dialect, variations in pitch and speed, and how distinct or slurred the pronunciation is. By filtering out acoustic events, which have no relevance for the current report, and making comparisons with known variations in speaker characteristics, the system can compensate for many of these deviations and normalize the speech for further processing. Next, the system must recognize what the speaker said. As with other challenges in speech recognition, the context – the probability model of words and word sequences – of the dictation is the key to generating high-quality and consistent results. This starts with vocabulary. Awareness of what people are likely to say not only helps recognize what they do say, it also helps identify what does not belong; for example, "PET" (positron emission tomography) is more likely in a radiologist's report than is "pet" (an animal kept at home). This awareness is also about knowing the probability of a particular word, given the words used before: the probability of "PET" being followed by "scan" is much higher than it being followed by "food".

Word Interpretation

Recognizing what was said provides a solid basis for correcting phrase and sentence structures. But spontaneous dictation often results in missing articles, verbs, and punctuation, as well as redundant or repeated words and self-corrections (Table 8). A clear understanding of the context helps interpretation of the words in order to identify and correct such matters.

Table 8. Examples of Word Interpretations and Situational Intelligence

	Dictated Text	Recognized Text
Redundant phrases	End of dictation. Thank you.	Does not appear in final document.
Redundant phrases	Send copy of report to	Does not appear in final document.
Section headings	Clinical Findings/History/ Section Next is section...	{Clinical History}
Dates	May five two thousand seven; fifth of May two thousand and seven; Five five ohh seven	May 5, 2007
Automatic punctuation	No chills fevers, night sweats, weight loss...	No chills, fevers, night sweats
Silences/pauses	There hasn't been (----pause----) much change...	There has not been much change.
Nonspeech dictation	There hasn't been (paper rustling) much change...	There has not been much change.
Hesitations	There hasn't been (AAHHMMMMM) much...	There has not been much...
Contraction	There hasn't been	There has not been

Controlling the Applications

The understanding of context also allows using speech recognition to control the user interface, a particularly attractive feature for doctors who prefer to look after the full report generation process. By differentiating command from dictation contexts, the speech recognition and word processing applications can be linked more closely to eliminate most of the remaining keyboard work. The doctor can open documents, switch on and off italics, go back and make corrections, spell unusual patient names, and so on, just using speech. For a radiologist, for example, this means being able to simultaneously dictate and manipulate an image. With some simple configuration, a doctor can even define personal "speech macros" with which to insert frequently used blocks of text or even to navigate through regularly used forms and fill them out completely, without a keyboard.

Rules and Analyses

Whether it is to dictate the content of a report or execute commands for the word processing application, the system works internally, with phonetic representations of words, and rules for the structures of phrases, sentences, and documents. The developers entered basic representations and rules, along with suitable vocabulary. The system then added more detail by statistically examining large numbers of existing texts. When transcribing dictation, the system compares the words on hand with these statistics to imply the word, phrase, sentence, or document section and adjusts the output accordingly.

Results

Speech recognition for dictation can be used for immediate production of reports by the clinician or as part of speeding up a traditional transcription service, allowing the transcriptionist or editor to concentrate on quality control – though obviously, the system helps here too, by getting the spellings right. Either way, it reduces the administrative overhead and shortens the time between dictation and report release, which many radiology departments appreciate, for example, to complement a PACS, which already accelerates the expectations of their colleagues elsewhere in the hospital. The bottom line is shorter patient waiting times and higher patient satisfaction.

Whatever the application, the heart of any speech-recognition system remains the intelligence that turns speech into text. By recognizing what is said, and interpreting it reasonably, ISI technology makes sure the transcription process requires the minimum of intervention to produce accurate reports.

Glossary

Accession number
Unique number assigned to an individual test or procedure by either the hospital information system (HIS) or radiology information system (RIS).

Acoustic adaptation
Process that continuously improves an author's acoustic references by analyzing dictation and automatically updating the acoustic reference file (ARF) to better understand an author's voice.

Context
The probability model of words and word sequences that contains the vocabulary (context lexicon) and the default language model for speech recognition. It contains words and word combinations, as well as information on pronunciation. Contexts are specific to one language and one field of application

DICOM
(Digital Imaging and COmmunications in Medicine)
A standard for interconnection of medical digital imaging devices developed by the American College of Radiology (ACR) and the National Electrical Manufacturers Association (NEMA). DICOM improves interconnectability of equipment on a network and interactivity with other communications standards.

PACS
(Picture Archiving and Communication Systems)
Systems that facilitate image viewing at diagnostic, reporting, consultation, and remote computer workstations, as well as archiving of pictures on magnetic or optical media using short- or long-term storage devices. PACS allow communication using local or wide-area networks, public communications services, systems that include modality interfaces, and gateways to health care facility and departmental information systems.

RIS
(Radiology Information System)
A system comprised of patient registration, film/chart tracking, scheduler, management reports, and other tools designed to increase the efficiency of radiology offices.

Suggested Readings

Amatayakul MK, Sattler AR. Computerization of the medical record – how far are we? *Fourteenth Annual Symposium on Computer Applications in Medical Care* 1990; 724-728

American College of Radiology. ACR Standard for communication: diagnostic radiology. In: Standards, Reston: *American College of Radiology*, 1995

American College of Radiology. Glossary of MR Terms, Reston, *American College of Radiology*, 1995

Barnhard HJ, Dockray KT. Computerized operation in the diagnostic radiology department. *Am J Roentgenol* 1970; 109:628-635

Barnhard HJ, Jacobson HG, Nance JW. Diagnostic radiology information system (DRIS). *Radiology* 1974; 14:314-319

Barnhard HJ, Lane GB. The computerized diagnostic radiology department: update 1982. *Radiology* 1982; 145:551-558

Barnhard HJ, Long JM. Computer autocoding, selecting and correlating of radiologic diagnostic cases. A preliminary report. *Am J Roentgenol* 1966; 96:854-863

Bell D, Greenes R. Evaluation of UltraSTAR: performance of a collaborative structured data entry system, *Proceedings of the 18th Annual Symposium on Computer Applications in Medical Care* 1994; 216-221

Bell D, Greenes R. Evaluation of UltraSTAR, performance of a collaborative structured data entry system, *J Am Med Inform Assoc* 1994; 216-222

Bell D, Greenes R, Doubilet P. Form-based clinical input from a structured vocabulary: Initial application in ultrasound reporting, *Proceedings of the 16th Annual Symposium on Computer Applications in Medical Care* 1992; 789-790

Bell D, Greenes R, Doubilet P. Form-based clinical input from a structured vocabulary: Initial application in ultrasound reporting. *J Am Med Inform Assoc* 1992; 789-791

Bell D, Pattison-Gordon E, Greenes R. Experiments in concept modeling for radiographic image reports. *J Am Med Inform Assoc* 1994; 1:249-262

Bell D, Pattison-Gordon E, Greenes R, Kahn C Jr. A conceptual-graph framework for structured reporting in radiology: application in pelvic ultrasound and breast imaging. In: Wolfman NT, Rowberg AH, eds. *Computer Applications to Assist Radiology*. Carlsbad: Symposia Foundation, 1994; pp 261-264

Berlin L. Comparing new radiographs with those obtained previously. *Am J Roentgenol* 1999; 172: 3-6

Berlin L. Communicating findings of radiological examinations: Whiter goest the radiologist's duty? *Am J Roentgenol* 2002, 178: 809-815

Berlin L. Duty to directly communicate radiologic abnormalities: has the pendulum swung too far? *Am J Roentgenol* 2003; 181:375-381

Berlin L. Standards, guidelines, and roses, *Am J Roentgenol* 2003; 181:945-950

Bernauer J. Conceptual graphs as an operational model for descriptive findings, *Proceedings of the Fifteenth Annual Symposium on Computer Applications in Medical Care* 1991; 214-218

Bernauer J, Gumrich K, Kutz S, Lindner P, Pretschner DP. An interactive report generator for bone scan studies. *Proceedings of the 15th Annual Symposium on Computer Applications in Medical Care* 1991; 858-860

Blais C, Samson L. The radiologic report: a realistic approach. *Can Assoc Radiolog J* 1995; 46:19-22

Bluth E, Havrilla M, Blakeman C. Quality improvement techniques: Value to improve the timeliness of preoperative chest radiographic reports. *Am J Roentgenol* 1993; 160:995-998

Brolin I. Systematisering och databehandling av rontgenutlatanden [Systematizing and data-processing X-ray reports], *Lakartidningen* 1967; 64:51-58

Brolin I. MEDELA: an electronic data-processing system for radiological reporting. *Radiology* 1972; 103:249-255

Brolin I. Radiologic reporting. I. Problems of structuring and coding information from diagnostic radiology. II. Medela reporting system. *Acta Radiologica* 1973; 323(Supplementum):1-151

Brolin I. Erfahrungen mit dem Medela-System [Experiences of the Medela system (author's transl)]. *Radiologe* 1974; 14:297-305

Campbell K, Musen M. Representation of clinical data using SNOMED III and conceptual graphs. *Sixteenth Annual Symposium on Computer Applications in Medical Care* 1992

Campbell KE, Wieckert K, Fagan LM, Musen MA. A computer-based tool for generation of progress notes. *Proceedings of the 17th Annual Symposium on Computer Applications in Medical Care* 1993; 284-288

Cascade PN, Berlin L. Malpractice issues in radiology. America College of Radiology standard for communication, *Am J Roentgenol* 1999; 173:1439-1442

Cavagna E, Berletti R, Schiavon F, Scarsi B, Barbaro G. L'ottimimizzazione dei tempi di consegna degli esami radiologici. La metodologia Six Sigma applicata ad una Unità Operativa di Radiodiagnostica. *Radiologica Medica* 2003; 105:205-214

Cavallo V, D'Aprile MR, Lanciotti S, Serianni L. Il referto radiologico e la sua leggibilità. *Radiologia Medica* 2001; 101:321-325

Cavallo V, Giovagnorio F, Messineo D, Volpe A. Proposta di un sistema originale di "input vocale mediato" nella refertazione radiologica. *Radiologia Medica* 1991; 82:738-740

Clayton P, Ostler D, Gennaro J, Beatty S, Frederick P. A radiology reporting system based oil most likely diagnoses *Comp Biomed Res* 1980; 13:258-270

Clinger N, Hunter T, Hillman B. Radiology reporting: Attitudes of referring physicians. *Radiology* 1988; 169:825-826

D'Orsi C, Kopans D. American College of Radiology's mammography lexicon: Barking up the only tree. *Am J Roentgenol* 1994; 162:595

Elmore JG, Wells CK, Lee CH, Howard DH, Feinstein AR. Variability in radiologists' interpretations; of mammograms. *New Engl J Med* 1994; 33:1493-1499

Freidman PJ. Radiologic reporting: structure. *Am J Roentgenol* 1983; 140:171-172

Gagliardi R. The evolution of the X-ray report. *Am J Roentgenol* 1995; 164:501-502

Gouveia-Oliveira A, Raposo V, Salgado N, Almeida I, Nobre-Leitao C, de Melo F. Longitudinal comparative study: The influence of computers on reporting of clinical data. *Endoscopy* 1991; 23:334-337

Greenes R. OBUS: A microcomputer system for measurement, Calculation, reporting, and retrieval of obstetric ultrasound examinations. *Radiology* 1992; 144:979-833

Greenes R, Barnett G, Klein S, Robbins A, Prior R. Recording, retrieval, and review of medical data by physician computer interaction. *New Engl J Med* 1970; 282:307-315

Hall FM. Language of the radiology report: primer for residents and wayward radiologist. *Am J Roentgenol* 2000; 175:1239-1242

Haugh PJ, Clayton PD, Tocino I, et al. Chest radiography: a tool for the audit of report quality. *Radiology* 1991; 180:271-276

Holman B, Aliabadi P, Silverman S, Weissman BN, Rudolph L, Fener U. Medical impact of unedited preliminary radiology reports. *Radiology* 1994; 191:519-521

Kahn C, Wang K, Bell D. Structured entry of radiology reports using world-wide web technology, *Radiographics* 1996; 16:683-691

Kalbhen C, Yetter E, Olson M, Posniak H, Aranha G. Assessing the resectability of pancreatic carcinoma: The value of reinterpreting abdominal CT performed at other institutions. *Am J Roentgenol* 1998; 171:1571-1576

Kong A, Barnett G, Mosteller F, Youtz C. How medical professionals evaluate expressions of probability. *New Engl J Med* 1986; 315:740-744

Kushner DC, Lucey LL. Diagnostic radiology reporting and communication: the ACR guideline. *J Am Coll Radiol* 2005; 2:15-21

Langlotz CP. Structured reporting in radiology. In: *Society for Health Service Research in Radiology*, Winter 2000, Newsletter

Langlotz CP. Automating structuring of radiology reports: harbinger of a second information revolution in radiology. *Radiology* 2002; 224:5-7

Leslie A, Jones AJ, Goddard PR. The influence of clinical information on the reporting of CT by radiologist *Br J Radiol* 2000; 73: 1052-1055

Magen A, Langlotz C, Banner M, Orel S, Sullivan D, Birnbaum B, Ramchandani P, Jacobs J. Interpretation of outside examinations: An undervalued service? Boston: *American Roentgen Ray Society* 1997

McLoughlin RF, So CB, Gray RR et al. Radiology reports: how much descriptive details is enough? *Am J Roentgenol* 1995; 165: 803-806

Melson D, Brophy R, Blaine J, Jost R, Brink G. Impact of a voice recognition system on report cycle time and radiologist reading time, In: Horii S, Blaine J, eds. *Proceedings of Medical Imaging* 1998

Horii S, Blaine J, eds. *Proceedings of SPIE Medical Imaging: PACS Design and Evaluation*, Bellingham: SPIE 1998:226-236

Moorman P, van Ginneken A, Siersema P, van der Lei J, van Bemmel J. Evaluation of reporting based on descriptional knowledge. *J Am Med Inform Assoc* 1995; 2:365-373

Musen M, Weickert K, Miller F, Campbell K, Fagan L. Development of a controlled medical terminology: Knowledge acquisition and knowledge representation. *Meth Info Mod* 1995; 34:85-95

Nishikawa RM, Doi K, Giger ML, Schmidt RA, Vyborny CJ, Monnier-Cholley L, Papaioannou J, Lu P. Computerized detection of clustered microcalcifications: Evaluation of performance on mammograms from multiple centers. *Radiographics* 1995; 15:443-452

Norman GR, Brooks LR, Coblentz CL, Babcook CJ. The correlation of feature identification and category judgements in diagnostic radiology. *Mem Cognit* 1991; 20:344-355

Pendergrass H, Greenes R, Barnett G, Poitras 1, Pappalardo A, Marble C. Ali on-line computer facility for systematized input of radiology reports. *Radiology* 1969; 92:709-713

Poon A, Fagan L, Shortliffe E. The Pen-Ivory project; Exploring user-interface design for the selection of items from large controlled vocabularies of medicine. *J Am Med Inform Assoc* 1996; 3:168-183

Revak CS. Dictation of radiologic reports (letter). *Am J Roentgenol* 1983; 141:210

Rogers LF. Information transfer: radiology reports, *Am J Roentgenol* 2001; 176:573

Rothman M. Malpractice issues in radiology: Radiology reports. *Am J Roentgenol* 1998; 170:1108-1109

Schiavon F, Berletti R. Il radiologo e la refertazione. Suggerimenti per una corretta comunicazione. Torino: *Edizioni Minerva Medica* 2006

Schiavon F, Berletti R, Guglielmi G, Cmmarota T. La diagnostica per immagini nell'invecchaimento. *Radiologia Medica* 2003; 106 (Suppl 1 al n. 3)

Schiavon F, Cavagna E, D'Andrea P, Carubia G. Immagini e parole. La tramissione delle immagini e la refertazione nella radiologia toracica (parte I). *Radiologia Medica* 2000; 99:223-232

Schiavon F, Cavagna E, D'Andrea P, Carubia G. Immagini e parole. La tramissione delle immagini e la refertazione nella radiologia toracica (parte II) *Radiologia Medica* 2000; 99:323-333

Schiavon F, D'Andrea P. Le attuali prestazioni radiologiche tra tecnologia, informazione, diagnosi e prevenzione. *Radiologia Medica*, in press

Schiavon F, Nardini S, Favat M, Vardanega A, Tregnaghi P. Problemi diagnostici nella lettura degli esami radiologici del torace di accoglimento dell'anziano. Esperienza personale. *Radiologia Medica* 1998; 96:48-54

Seltzer S, Kelly P, Adams D, Chiango B, Viero M, Fener E, Rondeau R, Kazanjian N, Laffel G, Shaffer K, Williamson D, Aliabadi P, Gillis A, Holman L. Expediting the turnaround of radiology reports: Use of total quality management to facilitate radiologists' report signing. *Am J Roentgenol* 1994; 162:775-781

Sobel J, Pearson M, Gross K, Desmond K, Harrison E, Rubenstein L, Rogers W, Kahn K. Information content and clarity of radiologists' reports for chest radiography. *Acad Radiol* 1990; 3:709-717

Steele JL, Nyce JM, Williamson KB, Gundermann RB. Learning to report. *Acad Radiol* 2002; 9:817-820

Swets JA, Getty DJ, Pickett RM, D'Orsi CJ, Seltzer SE, McNeil BJ. Enhancing and evaluating diagnostic accuracy. *Med Decis Making* 1991; 11:9-18

Tardáguila F, Martí-Bonmatí L, Bonmatí J. El informe radiologico: filosofía general (I), *Radiologia* 2004; 46(4):195-198

Tardáguila F, Martí-Bonmatí L, Bonmatí J. El informe radiologico: estylo y contenido (II). *Radiologia* 2004; 46(4):199-202

Tuddenham W. Glossary of terms for thoracic radiology; Recommendations of the Nomenclature Committee of the Fleischner Society. *Am J Roentgenol* 1984; 143:509-517

Vydareny KH. Radiology 1998: are today's residents ready for (tomorrow's) practice? *Am J Roentgenol* 1999; 173: 537-538

Subject Index

A

additional exam 28,29, 45, 48, 53, 55, 58, 60, 84
adults 85
ageing process 89
analysis 31, 44, 50, 52, 57, 72, 76, 82, 105, 117, 118
analytical report 50, 51
anomalies 97, 98
attention 17, 24, 51, 84, 91, 93-95, 98-100

B

borderline cases 86

C

certificate 27
children 85, 86, 101
chronic degenerative 41, 42, 44
clinical-anamnestic information 75
clinical data 45, 117
– request 29, 32, 57, 75-77, 82, 84, 106
– requirements images 3, 54
– suspicion 77, 79, 87
cognitive 18, 41, 92-96, 100
– errors 94, 96, 100
cognitive-ruled method 94
communication 1, 3, 19, 23, 24, 39, 49-51, 55, 56, 65, 66, 110, 113, 126
competence 25, 26, 66, 67
completeness 27, 34, 106

computer-assisted diagnosis (CAD) 7, 72
continuous 16, 110
control tests 47
cost-benefit 76
cost generators 83

D

diagnostic "puzzle" 29
– conclusion 28, 29, 83
– hypothesis 29
– requested 71
diagnosis combined 32
differential diagnostic 32, 112
digital technology 7, 79
direct signs 8, 71, 72
discreet 16, 66
document 1, 3, 27, 34, 91, 103, 105-108, 120-122, 125

E

effective 1, 23, 24, 26, 55, 56, 108, 110
elderly people 85-87, 89
emergency 98
equality 18, 19, 49
erroneous attribution 94
errors 2, 4, 50, 60, 75, 77, 91-101, 118, 120
ethical aspect 39
– sense 84
evidence-based medicine 3, 6, 80
execution 28, 30, 35, 73, 76, 82, 84